Praise for *Good Stress*

"Jeff Krasno is one of my favorite teachers and a truly wise guide for growth. Good Stress *beautifully reveals that so many of our stressors become our strengths. The grounded wisdom and actionable strategies make this a must-read for true well-being."*

— **Brendon Burchard**, #1 *New York Times* best-selling author of *The Motivation Manifesto* and *High Performance Habits*

"In Good Stress, *Jeff Krasno eloquently bridges the ancient wisdom of Eastern thought with modern scientific insights. This profound work reveals how Buddhist teachings on impermanence and interconnection anticipated groundbreaking discoveries in epigenetics, neuroplasticity, and the microbiome. This book is a masterful exploration of how embracing life's challenges can unlock our innate potential for growth, healing, and transformation."*

— **Deepak Chopra**, best-selling author of *The Seven Spiritual Laws of Success*

"Jeff's evolution from entrepreneur to author and thought leader embodies the transformative potential within each of us. In Good Stress, *he adeptly merges mysticism with medicine, presenting deep revelations on how embracing discomfort can catalyze authentic growth and healing. Jeff's prose serves as a poignant reminder that genuine wellness emerges not from evading challenges, but from boldly embracing them with fortitude and inquisitiveness. This book stands as a road map for individuals seeking to leverage the potency of 'good stress' to revolutionize their health, mindset, and overall life experience."*

— **Gabrielle Bernstein**, #1 *New York Times* best-selling author of *The Universe Has Your Back*

"In Good Stress, *my longtime friend Jeff Krasno takes us on an extraordinary journey from CEO to health advocate, blending wisdom from Eastern philosophy with the science of functional medicine. I've watched Jeff transform from a successful business leader at Wanderlust to a passionate storyteller who dives deep into the power of adversity mimetics. This book beautifully weaves ancient teachings on impermanence and interconnection with practical protocols that challenge the body and mind, showing us that true growth comes from embracing life's hard edges. It's a must-read for anyone ready to unlock the healing potential of 'good stress.'"*

— **Mark Hyman, M.D.**, co-founder and chief medical officer of Function Health and 15-time *New York Times* best-selling author

"This groundbreaking guide masterfully blends personal anecdotes, cutting-edge research, and practical protocols to help us reconnect with our biological roots. By adopting Krasno's deliberate short-term acute stress techniques, readers can unlock the evolutionary benefits that foster resilience and longevity. This transformative book is essential for anyone seeking to harness the power of 'in-convenience' to achieve optimal health and well-being."

— **David Perlmutter, M.D., F.A.C.N.**, #1 *New York Times* best-selling author of *Grain Brain* and *Drop Acid*

"In Good Stress, *Jeff Krasno masterfully illustrates the profound impact evolutionary mismatches have on our health and well-being. This book dives deep into the science of why our modern comfort-filled life, while seemingly benign, is at odds with our genetic makeup. With a focus on the transformative power of fasting—a topic near to my practice—and other eustress protocols, Jeff provides a compelling blueprint for realigning our lifestyle with our biology. This is not just a book; it's a call to action to embrace the stressors that refine us, challenge us, and ultimately lead us to a vibrant life. A must-read for anyone looking to break free from the grip of chronic ease and reclaim their health."*

— **Dr. Will Cole**, *New York Times* best-selling author of *Intuitive Fasting* and *Ketotarian*

"This book is a game-changer in understanding how to reclaim our health by embracing adversity. Having witnessed Jeff's transformation firsthand, I can attest to his commitment to mastering the science of the body—especially in the realm of blood sugar regulation and metabolic health. Jeff beautifully weaves together practical insights with deep wisdom, drawing on the same protocols we both use—intermittent fasting, cold plunging, sauna, and resistance training. Jeff's journey from pre-diabetes to vibrant health is inspiring, and this book offers a road map for anyone looking to harness the power of 'good stress' to thrive."

— **Dr. Sara Gottfried**, *New York Times* best-selling author of *The Hormone Cure* and leading expert in functional medicine

"Jeff Krasno masterfully delves into how embracing life's challenges can profoundly transform our health and well-being. As someone who has dedicated my life to teaching the power of growing your own food—specifically sprouting—I was thrilled to see Jeff spotlight this practice as a prime example of 'good stress.' The process of sprouting, especially broccoli sprouts, embodies the hermetic effect, where a little stress at the cellular level triggers powerful health benefits, including boosting our body's defenses and activating sulforaphane production. This book beautifully guides us back to our roots, to reconnect with nature, and reclaim our well-being. It's a must-read for anyone ready to tap into the life-changing benefits of doing hard things for a healthier, more vibrant future."

— **Doug Evans**, author of *The Sprout Book*

"In Good Stress, *Jeff Krasno deftly uncovers how modern culture has hijacked our biology, leading to a host of health challenges that stem from evolutionary mismatches. From the pitfalls of industrial agriculture to the dangers of sedentary living, temperature neutrality, and digital-only communication, Jeff provides a clear, science-backed road map for reclaiming our natural vitality. This book is an essential guide for anyone looking to realign their lifestyle with how we're truly wired, empowering us to harness the power of 'good stress' to become stronger, healthier, and more resilient."*

— **Jillian Michaels**, *New York Times* best-selling author of *Master Your Metabolism*

"Jeff Krasno brings a courageous approach to the most challenging conversations of our time. By applying the concept of adversity mimetics to healing our political divide, Jeff shows us that the discomfort of these dialogues can actually be a basis for growth, empathy, and the recognition of our shared humanity. This book is a profound reminder that facing our fears and moving through them can transform not only our personal lives but also our collective journey toward a more unified and compassionate society."

— **Marianne Williamson**, *New York Times* best-selling author of *A Return to Love*

"Good Stress *jumps off the pages as they are read. This book is like an experiential orgy of insights, experiences, and the tapestry of life's journey and how to live it. I thought that over the past fifty years in the health and wellness field that I had heard it all—until reading Jeff Krasno's masterpiece. This book not only takes you on a joyous trip but is capable of changing your perception of stress and making it your friend."*

— **Jeffrey Bland, Ph.D., FACN**, founder of the Institute for Functional Medicine

"Jeff has penned a vastly informed, dead-to-rights honest description of current health maladies, mysteries, and myths. He humorously and incisively walks a path that takes the reader to vitality and well-being, showing that a rebirth of our body and self is available to all."

— **Paul Hawken**, *New York Times* best-selling author of *Drawdown*

GOOD STRESS

ALSO BY JEFF KRASNO

Communion

Wanderlust

Wanderlust Find Your True Fork

GOOD STRESS

THE HEALTH BENEFITS OF DOING HARD THINGS

JEFF KRASNO

WITH SCHUYLER GRANT

HAY HOUSE INDIA
New Delhi • London • Sydney
Carlsbad, California • New York City

Hay House Publishers (India) Pvt Ltd
Muskaan Complex, Plot No. 3, B-2, Vasant Kunj, New Delhi – 110070, India

Hay House LLC, P.O. Box 5100, Carlsbad, CA 92018-5100, USA
Hay House UK Ltd, 1st Floor, Crawford Corner, 91-93 Baker Street, London W1U 6QQ, UK
Hay House Australia Publishing Pty Ltd, 18/36 Ralph St., Alexandria NSW 2015, Australia

Email: contact@hayhouse.co.in
Website: www.hayhouse.co.in

Indexer: J S Editorial, LLC
Cover design: The Book Designers
Interior design: Joe Bernier
Interior illustrations: Shayla Baylor

First published by Hay House India, 2025
10 9 8 7 6 5 4 3 2 1

ISBN 978-93-6611-233-6

Printed at Repro India Limited

MIX
Paper from responsible sources
FSC® C047271
FSC www.fsc.org

Hay House is committed to a sustainable future for our business, our readers and our planet. This book is made from Forest Stewardship Council® certified paper.

Dedicated to
my beloved estrogen footprint . . .
my daughters, Phoebe, Ondine, and Micah

CONTENTS

INTRODUCTION

Squeezing the Sponge

At the end of the end of the end of a road, nestled amid the undulating hills of the Santa Monica mountains, you will find Commune Topanga.

Actually, you will get very lost before you find it. The single-lane back roads will become progressively serpentine. You will drop all cellular service. Your heart rate will quicken at the precarity of the sheer cliffs dropping off the shoulder. You'll question your instincts and ask yourself why you agreed to travel to a remote retreat with no Internet called Commune.

Surely, you've seen enough documentaries about communes that don't end well.

For a brief moment, you will decelerate, maybe even pull over, and envision yourself kidnapped by a gaggle of naked hippies on acid. When this hesitancy inevitably occurs, you know you're very close to your destination, and, despite any lingering reticence, you press on.

Upon arriving, you may be met with a home-brewed kombucha or perhaps a tranche of warm seed bread. You settle into your rustic A-frame cabin—off the grid but nicely appointed with potted succulents. Slowly, your anxiety level drops along with your shoulders. Welcome to Commune.

Commune Topanga is our 10-acre experiment in well-being: one part production facility, one part retreat center, one part sustainability lab. There are meditation platforms perched above magical vistas, a crystal-laden yoga shala, glamping yurts, long communal dining tables, citrus and pomegranate groves, 14 honeybee hives, a peep of ISA Brown chickens, and an incessant trickle of fascinating people—like Scotty.

Scotty is the erstwhile head of waste management at Burning Man. Never has a man more enamored with human fecal matter walked the earth. Scotty installed an array of solar-powered compostable toilets on the property. Every few weeks, we help the decomposition process by feeding the bowl microbes. The microbes alchemize human scat into a potent compost tea. I wouldn't recommend it with milk and sugar, but the fruit trees love it. Little do they know, but as recurring visitors savor their apple crisp, they are unwittingly eating their own shit.

Schuyler, my long-suffering better three-quarters, and I have been manifesting this vision for decades. But lest you think it's paradise on earth, please know that septic is prone to backing up, ground squirrels often get to the lettuce before we do, and a bevy of bee stings once sent my Commune co-founder, Jake, into anaphylaxis. Be careful what you wish for.

I set this backdrop, for it is on this land that I have hosted and interviewed (and dined, hiked, cold-plunged, and sauna-bathed with) hundreds of the world's most prolific doctors, yogis, spiritualists, mystics, and sages. Yes, I have also played interlocutor in more prosaic settings on Zoom and in fluorescent-lit, dank-carpeted conference halls, but Topanga is where I have experienced the most profound moments of *satori*, absorbing the wisdom of so many diverse and facile minds in an environ that matches their singularity.

Over the past five years, since the launch of the *Commune Podcast*, I have paddled a conversational canoe with spiritual teachers like Deepak Chopra, Marianne Williamson, and Sadhguru. I have probed the mental gladstones of functional and integrative medicine physicians like Mark Hyman, Sara Gottfried, Jeffrey Bland, Zach Bush, Casey Means, Kara Fitzgerald, David and Austin Perlmutter, Jolene Brighten, and Terry Wahls. I've spoken with neuroscientists like Andrew Huberman and Adam Gazzaley, with nutritionists Elissa Goodman and Simon Hill, with environmentalists like Paul Hawken, Warren Brush, Finian Makepeace, Ryland Engelhart, and Kate Nelson and with trauma and addiction experts including Gabor Maté, Russell Brand, Hala Khouri, and David Kessler. I've jawed and nattered with purveyors of every bespoke wellness modality, including Wim Hof,

Byron Katie, Davidji, Tracee Stanley, Matteo Pistono, and Michael Beckwith, and with those who defy categorization like Matthew McConaughey, Mickey Hart, Marie Forleo, Jim Kwik, Dave Asprey, and Rener and Ryron Gracie. I could write another book about my madcap misadventures with these characters—but it would likely be my last.

In addition to interviewing living souls, I have spent hundreds of hours excavating the posthumous libraries of the British philosopher Alan Watts and the American spiritualist Ram Dass in collaboration with their estates. And, of course, I cohabitate with my Zen teacher and muse, Schuyler, whose iconoclasm serves me up daily koans over which to cogitate.

In preparation for the aforementioned interviews, I have read over 400 books, endless scientific papers, primary source data, and clinical research. If only out of vanity and risk of public embarrassment, I have committed myself to rigorous study, and, in doing so, I have become an "amateur everything," from citizen microbiologist to part-time Buddhist.

For years, I have had the unique opportunity to absorb the insight of the world's greatest minds. This book synthesizes and distills their wisdom into a guide for well-being—a coalescence of the ancient and the cutting edge. It is a squeezing of the sponge.

Why Write a Book?

I decided to write this book because I believe I have put my thumb on the amalgam of health protocols that can, as Dr. Mark Hyman quips, add not only years to our life but life to our years.

My discovery of these practices was propelled not only by curiosity but also by necessity. My health was teetering on the edge. What began as an intellectual inquiry quickly became a deeply personal journey. To my utter surprise, like most Americans, I was diagnosed with a chronic disease in 2018.

I ground much of this book in my own story, not because it's extraordinary, but, on the contrary, because it is so very ordinary. I didn't have Rasmussen's Encephalitis or Alice in Wonderland syndrome—both real conditions. I had brain fog and chronic fatigue, insomnia, and a jelly belly. Brown skin tags were budding in my armpits, and, worse, I developed ghastly fleshy protuberances on my chest (a.k.a. man boobs).

Subsequent to these unflattering physical presentations, I discovered that I was diabetic and had a leak in my gut.

My aforementioned symptoms are so common and prosaic in modern life that we've accepted them as normal. What people don't know is that metabolic dysfunction of the variety I was experiencing was, historically, as atypical as Stone Man syndrome, the world's rarest disease. But, now, 93 percent of Americans have metabolic dysfunction, a cluster of conditions that includes high blood pressure, high serum glucose, excess body fat around the middle, and abnormal cholesterol levels.[1] This syndrome is just upstream from modernity's Four Ubiquitous Contemporary Killers (yes, the FUCKs): heart disease, cancer, dementia, and diabetes.

As I peered despairingly into the mirror, futilely sucking in my substantial gut and flexing my non-extant pectorals, I asked myself: What is the provenance of all this disease? And how do we solve for it?

These questions prompted my own five-year inquiry into what begets real well-being, a journey that brought me directly to the protocols of Good Stress I will present in this book. These are the protocols that I adopted to reverse my onset of diabetes—one of the FUCKs—and that can be adopted by anybody who wants to recapture their agency over their healthspan and live a long and vital life.

My podcast research and conversations featured hundreds of health protocols. In response to this deluge of modalities and mushrooms, pills and praxes, I roused myself from the interview chair and became my own N-of-1 experiment. My mind and body and, dare I say, spirit became a laboratory for both the conventional and esoteric protocols of my interviewees.

Could I engage in holotropic breathwork as I froze in a 40-degree ice bath while on a 24-hour pomegranate fast as I gazed at a mandala? Could I do 50 nude air squats while pouring sweat in a sauna as I chanted Buddhist mantras?

I tried it all.

Sifting through the grifting was certainly part of the process. But, over the course of a few years, I autodidactically learned twice what I did in college.

Through the development and adoption of my Good Stress protocols, I was able to reverse my diabetes and insulin resistance while also losing 60 pounds. I was the chubby kid that couldn't do one pull-up. Today, I do 20 at a time. Not long ago, the notion of reading an entire book, let alone writing one, was inconceivable. I have reclaimed my capacity to concentrate among the pings and dings of modernity. Once prone to mentally drifting away from a conversation, I now gift people the present of presence. I can already presage the eyerolls of my daughters as they read this paragraph, and I surely remain a world apart from my best self, but I am healing—moving toward wholeness. And you can too.

Why Are We Sick?

Our epidemic of chronic disease should actually be no surprise. It is the natural and expected by-product of our paleolithic genome trying to cope with our modern lifestyle. Our current collection of infirmities is a result of our overdependence on what I call the Big MACs (big modern American conveniences). While America has no monopoly on creature comforts, it certainly leads the way.

Over the past century, culture has evolved primarily for ease and convenience, resulting in an overabundance of highly processed calories, sedentariness, temperature neutrality, indoor living, near total reliance on digital devices, increased social isolation, and a perpetual drip of cortisol-dysregulating blue light from our omnipresent screens.

In the pages ahead, I will explain how these artifacts of modernity directly lead to obesity, depression, sleep disruption, and the panoply of our current epidemics.

It is our culture of "chronic ease" that is leading directly to the scourge of chronic *dis*-ease. In short, the way we live creates evolutionary mismatches. Humans evolved over millennia to thrive in conditions where discomfort and stressors were the norm. Our modern lifestyle hijacks our biology and renders our hard-wrought adaptive mechanisms maladaptive.

But there is a way to counteract this chronic ease.

Acute short-term Good Stress in the human body confers a health benefit and activates pathways that promote longevity and resilience. This phenomenon is called hormesis. On a biological level, we are just not engineered for lives of uber-convenience, and now we are paying the price. Adopting the protocols of Good Stress is therefore how we bring our bodies that have been ravaged by our reliance on the Big MACs back into balance.

You may be thinking that you are already awash in stress and wondering why you'd choose more. But, as I will untangle, there is a gargantuan difference between modern "chronic" stress and good "eustress."

What Is Good Stress?

Good Stress is my curated program of deliberate short-term acute stress protocols that realign us with our biology. Good Stress distills all my conversations, research, and self-experimentation into a unique consolidated program that unwinds the pathologies of chronic "ease."

Periods of calorie restriction due to food scarcity, exposure to extreme heat and cold, early morning light therapy, manual labor, connection to nature, face-to-face communication, and living in community were simply part of life for tens of thousands of years.

We evolved in relation to these paleolithic, and sometimes harsh, environmental conditions. These stressors, as I will explain, activated longevity pathways and built resilience. But, now, in an era of uber-convenience, we need to purposefully self-impose these conditions as a means to be well. Through the adoption of paleolithic stressors, which I sometimes call the protocols of "inconvenience," we leverage our inherent engineering. We swim with nature's current.

As you will read, my Good Stress program takes deliberate adversity beyond merely the physical. I extrapolate on physiological stressors and apply them to other essential components of well-being that have been eroded by modernity, including both psychological and social wellness. My mind training praxes help us wrest back our concentration spans from the "attention" economy. In an era of increasing loneliness, my *social* fitness regimen actively helps to foster the human connections that are essential to being well. I also share how absorbing insult built my "psychological immune system" and helped regulate my emotional vacillations.

In the chapters ahead, I will share my experiences of Good Stress. I unpack the practices, the science behind them, their often mystical roots, their conferred and often surprising benefits, and their recommended dosages.

My goal here is to combine my personal, at times comical, story with expert commentary and hard science to help you understand how to realign with your evolutionary advantages that nature has engineered to foster homeostasis—balance in the human body.

Book Anatomy

While I've included a significant amount of geeky medical science in this book, I both defer and refer to the people with letters after their name. I am more poet than physician. Hence, while I stress the importance of understanding mechanism, my descriptions of physiological processes are meant to entertain as much as educate, to teach through story and metaphor (and a smattering of regrettable dad jokes) as well as exposition and peer-reviewed studies. Hopefully, it will provide a reprieve from the Vesuvius of sanctimony that is the signature of the "wellness industry."

Yes, this book will absolutely provide my actionable Good Stress protocols which, if adopted, will usher you into greater well-being. However, while I will plumb the depths of fasting, exercise and light, and heat and cold-water therapies—all of which are wonderful protocols in the right circumstances—I am prescribing more than just a script. I am striving to provide a broader way of understanding well-being.

This book is organized into two distinct, interconnected sections. Essentially, in Part I, I describe what wellness is, and then, in Part II, I prescribe how to actually be well.

Part I outlines the four philosophical principles that underpin Good Stress: impermanence, interdependence, agency, and balance. I think of this as prepping the soil before you grow the veggies. It outlines a broader, at times mystical, framework for understanding well-being—as if Alan Watts, between refilling tumblers of vodka, penned a book on health. It overturns numerous core assumptions of who we think we are. We have been taught to think we are fixed, isolated individuals with predetermined fates controlled by our genes. However, both modern medicine and Eastern thought converge to point us in a very different direction. We have entered a new "age of agency"—a new paradigm in which we play an active part in cultivating the balance that leads to health.

Who the heck cares about philosophy? Well, philosophy, or the love of wisdom, is an activity people undertake when they seek to understand fundamental truths about themselves and their relationship to the world. Philosophy can, at times, be difficult to comprehend and even frustrating when you just want someone to tell you *what to do* to be healthy. If you just want the protocols, skip the pablum and go directly to Part II. Don't pass Go and don't collect $200. However, consider that understanding foundational truths about the nature of your organism will serve as the compost from which the garden of your well-being will flourish.

Part II outlines my specific Good Stress protocols that, if adopted, will foster balance and well-being. I will outline their modes of action, their benefits, and what to do. I examine the evolutionary mismatches caused by rapid changes in culture and how our modern lifestyle has upended many of our adaptive mechanisms.

To make our journey more enjoyable, I introduce my distant hunter-gatherer ancestor, Ffej Onsark, as a means to elucidate humanity's hard-wrought adaptations. By describing the "stressful" environment in which Ffej and hundreds of generations before and after him survived and thrived, I unpack the evolutionary adaptations that emerged across massive swaths of time.

To paraphrase Nietzsche, what didn't kill Ffej made him stronger. Food paucity, strenuous physical activity, exposure to the sometimes harsh vicissitudes of nature, and communal living activated pathways of longevity and resilience. In order to reap the same benefits, we now must deliberately self-impose these conditions. Good Stress helps us live a little more like Ffej.

ACKNOWLEDGMENTS

In elevator-pitching this book, I have often resorted to this description: imagine if Alan Watts and Dr. Mark Hyman had a baby. This book is an effort to midwife this progeny—in a literary sense.

While Watts didn't speak much to medicine, he did hint at the microbiome nearly 50 years before the concept entered the zeitgeist. It is Watts's broader understanding of Eastern mysticism and the intelligence of nature that has broad applicability to human physiology, and, ultimately, well-being.

Of course, I do not contend, though I occasionally pretend, to have the eloquence of Watts, whose essence perfumes this book on every page. I do aspire to his jocular mode of communication, which lives on as compellingly today as it did 50 years ago. His profound understanding of the course of nature anchors my understanding of human physiology in the mystical realm.

Mark Hyman is a brilliant functional medicine doctor whom I have known for many years. While functional medicine is on the cutting edge of Western science, it also rests atop many of the precepts of ancient Eastern thought. Little known fact: Mark was an Eastern religions major as an undergraduate. He also initially introduced me to many of the adversity mimetics (which I have dubbed Good Stress protocols) that I unpack in this book.

The more I studied Watts's metaphysical noodlings on impermanence, interdependence, and the unity of opposites, the more I saw it patterned everywhere in the physical human body. Hence, this book attempts at junctures to bridge the mystical and the medical.

I would be remiss to not acknowledge both Dr. Casey Means and Dr. Sara Gottfried, who have chaperoned me through a massive learning curve. I used to quake at the sight of a white coat, and now I want to wear one—provided it's nicely fitted. Their influence and tutelage on all things metabolic and hormonal have been inestimable. Deep gratitude as well to Gabor Maté, who has long explored the overlap between Buddhism and medical science and has generously provided guidance on many topics.

This book also draws significant inspiration from Fritjof Capra and his masterpiece, *The Tao of Physics*, in which the physicist articulates the convergence between the intuitive knowledge of Eastern religions and the empirical knowledge of 20th-century physics. This book builds upon the shoulders of Capra to further elucidate how many of his refrains apply to medical science and, ultimately, to the pursuit of well-being.

I extend my deep gratitude to my Commune team and partners, particularly my co-founders Jake Laub and Austin Rettig, who have generously provided me with the space to pen this book. I also harbor a boatload of appreciation for Chandrima Ornvold, Matteo Pistono, and Komal Yadav for their insightful contributions and essential edits. And I send a robust meow of recognition to my agent, Kitty, who accepts nothing less than purr-fection.

I am also profoundly thankful for the team at Hay House publishing, including Reid Tracy and Patty Gift, for believing that I have something valuable to contribute to the world's bank of ideas, and for my editor, Anne Barthel, for indulging my loquacity and rendering this book heaps better that it would have otherwise been.

And lastly, but certainly not leastly, I owe a great debt to my childhood, middle-aged (and hopefully old-aged) sweetheart, Schuyler. She, of course, reminds me of this liability on a quotidian basis. Without her, I'd likely be 400 pounds, day-drinking in a dive bar betting my last nickel on horses at Belmont. Schuyler gallantly fulfills so many roles in my life, including lover, teacher, muse, and, more than likely one day, nurse. There is so much to be grateful for, but my deepest appreciation lies here: Schuyler allows me to take outlandish risks and pursue wild dreams, knowing that, in failure, I always have the soft, if slightly stained, pillow of her unconditional love to cushion the fall.

Working with her on this book has been equal parts delight and displeasure. For it *is* work. I'm huffing through her yoga class and then writing about it as beads of sweat splatter the keyboard, only to receive a document from her the next morning brimming with red ink. Schuyler suffers no fools—including me. She is straightforward and unafraid to ruffle feathers. True to her character, she has applied a meat cleaver to this book and tenderized it like she does a flank steak—grass-fed, of course. As a result, this book is both more flavorful and easier to digest.

Schuyler has made me better for 36 years, and this collaboration is no exception. In remuneration, I have dutifully delivered three X chromosomes. I suppose you could consider this book our fourth daughter. Let us hope it doesn't require a diaper change.

A NOTE FROM SCHUYLER GRANT

Long-term relationships are a compendium of various myths compiled in partnership. These stories are reified day after day, year after year, and eventually feel like incontrovertible fact. Even more than the stories we tell ourselves about ourselves, the stories we reinforce about each other carry particular weight. Pun intended.

Jeff and I met in college and married in our mid-20s, and one of the foundational "truths" in the story of our marriage was that I won the genetic lottery—in the metabolism department anyway. Jeff's Eastern European ticket might have conferred a bounty of brain power, but, the story went, he inherited the "thrifty gene" from his Jewish side. And the truth was, I could eat just about the same amount of food as he could and I'd stay relatively thin and he would put on a pound or two just by looking askance at a bagel and schmear.

Undoubtedly, I come from a family of generally thin and health-conscious people. I grew up on a small hippie farm in Northern California, a most advantageous environment for setting up a healthy microbiome. I ate a lot of dirt. My mom was a food fascist and, though I binged on Oreos and Cap'n Crunch at my friends' houses whenever possible, my intake of processed foods was minimal. Besides a history of lower back pain, for my first four decades, I was the healthiest person I knew. Zippy metabolism aside, I simply never got sick. (Aside from going to the doctor one time when I was run over by a VW bus at age 2, I didn't see the inside of a doctor's office or hospital until I was 40 years old. This is not an exaggeration.)

Jeff's upbringing was pretty average, which means pretty SAD (standard American diet). Not a food desert by any stretch of the imagination, but plenty of processed foods and not enough soil microbes. He was a chubby kid, who got his skinny on by the time I met him at 17, and then he swung on the weight pendulum for decades. It was almost impossible for him to put on muscle and there was a cushion that encased his body—especially around his belly and legs. (I sometimes remarked to myself that his ass and thighs were more womanly than mine. Not a compliment to either of us.) But the issues went beyond what frankly sounds pretty superficial as I write this. Chronic insomnia and a depressed immune system were the most debilitating of the deeper level of his systemic dis-ease.

Nature vs. nurture? It's difficult, probably impossible, to untangle. But Jeff rewrote this thread of our narrative, through sheer force of will.

After three decades of building a life and a codependent story together, Jeff set out on an autodidactic health quest that provided the impetus for this book. I will let him elaborate on all the specifics and more. But what I can attest to is how shocking and awe-inspiring it was to witness the transformation of someone's health. Up close and very personal. It wasn't so much that Jeff lost 50 pounds, it was that he rewired his body. It was surreal to watch it happen. It wasn't that he lost fat around his ass and legs—it was a complete transformation of the shape of his body and the makeup of his cells. And he wasn't exactly a spring chicken when he set out to incubate and hatch his new self.

As you will learn, this journey began in the depths of pandemic lockdown. Jeff was hit with a one-two punch of Covid. He was first taken down in February of 2020, before we even knew that SARS-CoV-2 had made it into the U.S. But it was the second round a few months later that really clubbed him. He was not just sick, but very sick. And it went on a long, long time, before we even knew there was such a thing as "long Covid."

I got a small sniffle. It must have been really annoying.

But out of the proverbial mud of illness and upheaval, Jeff's intellectual lotus began to flourish. This was to be the beginning of Jeff's triumph over physical tribulation, his adventures in hormesis.

He began studying, and writing, and then experimenting—primarily on himself. We were lucky enough to shelter in place in a most special place: our small retreat property in Topanga Canyon, where we scrambled to pivot digital iterations of our work selves, while keeping our three daughters (aged 10 to 15 at the time) from losing their minds. I was forced to forgo my Luddite ways and bring my NYC yoga studio online; Jeff took on the challenge of penning a weekly newsletter, where he interrogated the nuances of the unfolding pandemic, from both a scientific and a sociological perspective. I naturally fell into the role of his editor. The world outside and inside continued to provide ample fodder for Jeff's literary probing. He poked and prodded at everything from the societal underpinnings of BLM to the intersectionality between Alan Watts and Niels Bohr. I nipped and tucked and prodded his prose.

I remember in my teens reading a passage from Anais Nin about love being a dance between the lover and the beloved. A bird and a hand. This struck me as true before I even knew it was true. Now, having done the hard work of a multidecade partnership, I firmly believe that in the healthiest relationships partners trade this dynamic back and forth. A similar, if less romantic, ingredient to a functional partnership is the ability to cosplay the role of the supporter and the supported.

Two decades ago, when we turned off the road of duo into the wilderness of parenthood, I was largely driving the bus. I had very firm opinions about how to have a baby (at home) and how to raise those babies (no parenting books required). Jeff graciously, if somewhat reluctantly, schlepped to home birth classes with Ina May Gaskin, blew up the birthing tub, and navigated the skeptical grandparents. He didn't eat the placenta, but he helped hydrate and encapsulate it. He co-slept and slung the babies around Brooklyn and let me navigate the vaccine schedules and homeschool co-ops.

Twenty years later it was my turn to undergird Jeff's creative process and four years of intellectual gestation. His unsatiable curiosity, his N-of-1 experimentation, a healthy dose of his irrepressible wit, and my midwifery have now produced another offspring. This book.

To be honest, when Jeff and I first met, he was a monosyllabic, banjo-picking pothead. Yes, he had gotten into Columbia, so he clearly wasn't a dummy, and he was undoubtedly easy on the eyes, but I thought I might be better suited to more of a conversationalist. Now 35 years later, I can't get the guy to shut up. All I wanna do is sit in bed and stream something on Netflix and he wants to geek out together about ATP and cellular function.

The lesson here might be . . . be careful what you ask for. It took a while, but now I have a super ripped hubby who won't shut up. And because Newtonian logic rules our households as well as the wider universe, for every domestic action there is an equal and opposite reaction. So now I am eating cookies and drinking wine for two. But there's a book I could recommend, which would inspire me to up my game a notch or two—or ten. And here it is. . . .

PART I

THE PRINCIPLES OF GOOD STRESS

What Is Well-Being?

CHAPTER 1

THE DREAM

(. . . and the Nightmare)

It is not true that people stop pursuing dreams because they grow old, they grow old because they stop pursuing dreams.

— Gabriel García Márquez

The Dream

The year is 2088. I am 118 years old, and my beloved Schuyler and I are celebrating a century together.

The afternoon is warm, and Schuyler and I hike up the canyon trail as we've done hundreds of times. We walk and talk, and talk and walk, getting lost in each other. Our fingers tickle the leaves of the madrones and the California peppers and the desert willows. Schuyler massages a fistful of French lavender between her palms and cups her creased hands over my nose. I inhale deeply. Her fingers are redolent with the flower's evergreen, woodsy perfume.

We arrive at our summer cabin and unpack our provisions. We'll prepare our favorite dinner—a cedar-smoked salmon, a sautéed lemon-zested spinach, and some roasted yams.

Schuyler gathers herbs from the garden to garnish the meal. Herbs are all we can manage to cultivate, but still the sage, the rosemary, and the oregano are abundant. They grow almost on their own.

I uncork a bottle of Chateau Margaux, one that we've been saving. We breathe with it languorously. As its flavor unwinds and tannins soften, so do we. We sip—thimble by thimble—as we dice garlic and shallots, thinly slice the sweet potatoes, and flash-grill the fish.

We glance at one another with present moment nostalgia. Our eyes tell each other that "these are the good old days."

After dinner, we wander into the twilight, out onto the porch, and drink in the cooled high-desert air. Schuyler takes my hand and leads me back to the bedroom. We make a kind of love—not with the unbridled passion of our youth. When we were teenagers, we actually necked, barefoot and fully recumbent, on the sidewalk of Amsterdam Avenue. No, this is a gentle, if slightly languid, kind of lovemaking. The yin and yang tattoos that we got when we were 17 on our respective breasts yoke into an ultimate, if wrinkly, unified reality.

And then she reads to me from the same interminable *New Yorker* article on plate tectonics that we'll never finish. Hearing the hushed parasympathetic breath of my impending slumber, she flips the brass dolly switch on the reading lamp. The world goes dark. She spoons me. And we drift off.

Sometime in the middle of the night, in the depths of slow-wave sleep, the mitochondria in my neurons and in my cardiac cells and the mitochondria in her neurons and her cardiac cells gradually reduce production. Our energy factories produce one last plume of carbon dioxide out their chimneys. Our roles as links in a continuous chain of captured sunlight come to a close. This life, the way we've known it, returns to the silence from whence it came. Schuyler and I float outside the vacillations of time, space, location, and form. In our sleep, our lives become rounded by a greater one. And it's okay. It's completely okay.

One night, more than a half century back, after reading a dozen fairy tales to our daughter Micah, she asked me, "If you were a prince and had one wish, what would it be?" I whispered back to her, "Well, I am a prince, and I wish that one day, a long time from now, your mother and I will die on the same day." Being closer to spirit, she immediately understood that this wish was not in the least morbid.

The following morning, our girls arrive dutifully at the cabin. Phoebe, Ondine, and Micah carefully wrap us up like tamales in burial shrouds of palm fronds. They wheel us out into the pasture that cascades down from the cottage and plant us among the wild grasses, buckwheats, and clovers. This ritual represents the only courteous thing to do. Given how much energy we have extracted from the planet, now it's time to donate all our carbon, nitrogen, calcium, phosphorus, sulfur, potassium, sodium, and magnesium back from whence it came, to play our part in nature's reciprocity. With the help of mycelium and fungi, our organisms will gracefully decay. Microbes and earthworms will feast away, metabolizing our bodies into rich, moist, black soil.

Near our interment, our daughters plant two acorns, perhaps a little closer together than an expert arborist might advise. Every summer, when the girls and their broods come visit, they can watch us grow as they read and rock on the front porch. From acorn, to sprout, to seedling, to plant, to tree laden with acorns and around again. Eventually, our upper branches will tangle, our trunks will gnarl and fuse, our understory becoming one. And, someday, our family will make a grove.

Admittedly, this might all sound a little maudlin. It's perhaps Pollyanna to think that death could be so unproblematic and effortless. But it's equally absurd that our expiration should have to entail 20 years of dialysis, statins, insulin injections, and worse.

Of course, the real dream is that the dream is not a dream.

Our true collective fantasy is that our healthspan becomes equal to our lifespan. That we can, as Dr. Mark Hyman proposes, "die young at an old age." That we not only add years to our life but also life to our years. However, the reality for the overwhelming majority of modern humans more resembles a nightmare than a fairy tale in a mountain cabin.

The Nightmare

For all the talk in the popular media about longevity, you might be surprised to know that, over the 7 years between 2014 and 2021, life expectancy actually declined 2.8 years in the United States from 78.9 to 76.1. This downward trend began well before COVID-19 put its wicked foot to the gas.

More problematic than the decrease in average solar orbits per capita (lifespan) is the average duration of our underlying "healthspan," the period of life spent in good health, free from the chronic diseases and disabilities of aging. In the modern West, life expectancy has become concomitant with "sick expectancy."

Sixty percent of Americans suffer from at least one chronic disease, the four most prevalent and deadly of which are cardiovascular disease, cancer, diabetes, and dementia.[1] I dub these the Four Ubiquitous Contemporary Killers (yes, the FUCKs).

And 40 percent are managing multiple chronic conditions, including other insidious characters such as non-alcoholic fatty liver disease (NAFLD), stroke, kidney disease, and depression.[2] The number rises to 80 percent in people aged 65 and over.[3] And, if you've made it to 80, on average, you have five chronic diseases. The average American spends the final 16 years of their existence limping through life, experiencing a reverse alchemy in which our golden years are converted to the base metals of wheelchairs and bedpans.

This epidemic of disease has myriad knock-on impacts. None of them good. Obviously, there is the pain, decrepitude, immobility, and cognitive decline that must be endured by the individual. This suffering then radiates out to friends and family members who must provide care, sometimes over decades, to infirmed loved ones. Additionally, there is the staggering societal expense. America currently spends $4.5 trillion on "sick" care, approximately 18 percent of total GDP,[4] primarily treating the symptoms of preventable chronic diseases with cocktails of pharmaceutical drugs. If the trajectory continues apace, domestic health care expenditures will increase to $10 trillion per year by 2040 and threaten to bankrupt the economy.[5]

Further, the distension of morbidity has eroded the value that was once attributed to accumulated experience. Older people were once heralded as fonts of wisdom. Now, our elders have become the *elderly*. Once revered for their insight, the old are now too often considered a nuisance and cast off to a facility. Can you imagine Confucius being shipped off to a nursing home?

There is also an oft-neglected political dimension to the chronic disease epidemic. Inflammation in the individual body is spilling over into the body politic. The current divisive and sickly political invective that dominates the world stage is a direct reflection of a population that is increasingly unwell. Currently, the obesity rate in the United States is 44 percent, with 11 percent of the country morbidly obese.[6] While being overweight is not always a reflection of poor underlying metabolic health, obesity is often both a cause and a symptom of metabolic dysfunction and associated with a panoply of pathologies.

Increasingly, science is demonstrating that physiological disease is interconnected with mental disorders. The scourge of mental conditions including, but not limited to, depression, autism, ADHD, OCD, PTSD, addiction, schizophrenia, bipolar disorder, and dementia are now estimated to impact one in every five Americans of all ages. There is mounting evidence that mental conditions and neurodegenerative diseases are, in some part, metabolic disorders.

The root causes of chronic disease, as I will elucidate in this book, are largely by-products of our lifestyle. In essence, in the modern world, we're not dying from infection and the communicable diseases that riddled human history. On the contrary, today we are choosing the way we die—and not with tremendous thoughtfulness.

Our escalating rates of illness should not be in the least surprising. During a recent interview in Topanga, Gabor Maté shared this analogy from high school biology class. Remember when you put a bacterial cell in a petri dish? If you fed the agar with some delectable carbon and nitrogen and maintained a proper temperature, then you would expect the bacterial cell to proliferate. If you, on the contrary, added caustic compounds like alcohol or bleach, the expectation would be very different. The cell would become dysfunctional and die.

The biological medium of a petri dish is called a culture.

If you put a person in a toxin-free culture of nutrient-rich food, safety, and abundant nature, then you would expect that individual to develop healthfully. If you put that person in a culture of ultra-processed foods and sugars, incessant stress, fear, neglect, and toxicity, then a physiologically and psychologically diseased person is a normal result.

The origins of our chronic disease epidemic are slightly more nuanced. While I poked at this notion in the introduction, this core concept bears repeating as it is so central to the etiology of our problem. The chronic illnesses that are plaguing society are not "bugs in the system." They are the natural and expected by-products of dependence on the Big MACs.

Dating back to the Industrial Revolution and accelerating over the last 50 years, culture has evolved primarily for ease and convenience. Modern agriculture produces a surfeit of nutrient-deficient cheap calories. "Convenience" stores hawk this foodstuff on every block. Digital thermometers maintain a constant controlled temperature in our living spaces. High-speed Internet, on-demand entertainment, and social media have become a form of mass hypnosis. Easy chairs, comfy shoes, and indoor living have cleaved humans from their natural habitat. These artifacts of modernity have deadly downstream impacts.

Chronic *dis*-ease is the direct result of a culture of chronic ease. Simply put, humans evolved over millennia to thrive in conditions where stress and discomfort were normal. Acute short-term stress in the human body confers a health benefit and activates pathways that promote longevity and resilience. On a biological level, we are simply not engineered for lives of uber-convenience, and now we are paying the price.

The nightmare of chronic disease is insidious and furtive in nature. It does not come on like the Texas chainsaw murderer. It unfolds slowly like a French film noir. Chronic disease slithers like a snail, moving so slowly that you don't even notice it. The FUCKs take hold sinisterly and develop sluggishly and progressively. They take root in your 20s and 30s and present initially in the most prosaic of ways: brain fog, fatigue, irritability, the inability to concentrate, disrupted sleep. Slowly, and then all of a sudden, you have diabetes or cancer, or, even worse, are struck down suddenly by myocardial infarction.

Fifty percent of Americans currently have diabetes or prediabetes.[7] Of those with prediabetes, 90 percent are unaware of their condition.[8] Like 100 million Americans, I was in the nightmare, ostensibly FUCK'd, and I didn't even know it.

CHAPTER 2

WELLTH & HELLNESS

How I Got Here

We become the stories we tell ourselves.

— Michael Cunningham

My introduction to wellness began rather incongruously with the attack on the World Trade Center. My business partner, Sean, and I were running an independent record label just two blocks north of what became Ground Zero. After the tragedy in 2001, our office was inaccessible for months, cordoned off within the tight perimeter of the cleanup area. When we did finally return to our Warren Street office, it was a mess. Soot everywhere. People nowhere. Our office building was for all intents and purposes abandoned.

Newton's third law of motion posits that for every action there is an equal and opposite reaction. Applying this axiom to life, colossal events can sometimes inspire commensurate outsized responses. This was certainly true for Schuyler. Out of the ashes of 9/11, Schuyler decided to open a yoga studio on the vacant floor above our office. The studio launched in early 2002 with a handcrafted street-side sandwich board promising "spirituality through sweat," and it quickly became a place of refuge for the beleaguered denizens of Lower Manhattan.

This was no multistory Equinox, mind you. Schuyler's shala predated the era of ubiquitous tony yoga studios and fitness centers. The studio was pre-Lycra funky with a bathroom the width of a bread box and a whistling radiator that set the tonic for the oms that bookended class. Schuyler called the studio "a community enterprise" and named it appropriately Kula Yoga Project. *Kula* translates to "intentional community" in Sanskrit.

A hundred times, I climbed up the cockeyed lime-green steps from my office to Kula to witness the same scene. Sweaty, blissed-out yoginis circled up post-class in the minute vestibule. They lingered—open-hearted, engaged, sometimes laughing, mostly crying, nursing each other back to sanity.

This was my first taste of the power of yoga and community to heal.

In the following years, as Schuyler began to lead retreats to the Osa Peninsula of Costa Rica, I bumped along on dozens of trips in the name of yoga. In all candor, I mostly avoided the actual practice, but I was entranced by the scene. Millennials, mostly women, a smattering of gay men, and me communed in the jungle—waking with the sun, surfing, meditating, practicing asana, cooking from the garden, and sharing the stories of our broken and remembered lives. But there was very little New Age sanctimony to it. Folks drank just enough wine and tequila at night and there were plenty of titillating illicit hookups. Far from the humdrum comforts of dull care, these yogis and yoginis gathered in the jungle to tap into a more vibrant and inspired life.

It was there, sequestered deep in the rainforest of Costa Rica, that I had the idea for Wanderlust. What if, I wondered, we could create the world's biggest yoga retreat? I now reflect on what an utterly male idea that was.

It wasn't a straight line, but that's exactly what we did. We took the essence of what Schuyler created in Costa Rica and produced it through the lens of Lollapalooza. We celebrated yoga teachers and meditation instructors as if they were Radiohead and Coldplay, putting them on big stages with booming sound systems and fancy light rigs. We mounted these transformational festivals on mountainsides across North America. It was a magnificent, grueling, life-bending endeavor. At its peak, we produced 68 full-scale events in 20 countries, drawing hundreds of thousands of people.

For a decade, Wanderlust became my entire life. I worked 16 hours per day, seven days a week. My travel schedule was insane and I rarely slept. Naively, we took on private equity investors. Their edict was simple: grow! But the money didn't come for free. These cigar-smoking plutocrats, perched atop a glass Midtown panopticon, scrutinized our every move.

Wanderlust consumed me, and eventually it expelled me out its anus like insoluble fiber. For 10 years, I helped keep the company "regular." But my lofty pursuits in health and wellness had somewhere along the line taken a sharp turn into the depths of "wellth and hellness."

In 2018, I exited Wanderlust—somewhat suddenly and acrimoniously. After my departure, I spiraled into a depression. I suffered from wicked insomnia. I spent countless nights brooding, plotting revenge schemes against our investors, holding resentment's ember in my palm, waiting for the right time to throw it. Of course, all this time, it was me who was getting burned.

While my brain galloped like a racehorse at night, it moped like a donkey during the day. I couldn't focus. I was sluggish. Brain fog and chronic fatigue became my default state. Coffee-fueled mornings and wine-filled evenings didn't help my cause. I thought I could mitigate my petty vices by going to the gym. But a half-hearted hour on the treadmill kept me just there . . . trudging along the treadmill of life half-heartedly.

I didn't appear all that ghastly. I camouflaged the bags under my eyes with tortoiseshell Ray-Bans and the inner tube around my middle with shapeless XL J. Crew button-downs. But I was tipping the scale at 206. I kept hurting my lower back and pulling my calf muscles.

Mostly, I was just tired.

It wasn't until I slapped a continuous glucose monitor on my triceps that I got a bucket of cold water over my head—which, at this juncture, was not a deliberate self-imposed protocol. A continuous glucose monitor (or CGM) is a disk-like sensor that one can apply to observe one's blood glucose levels. The sensor links neatly with an app and provides the wearer with a window into their metabolic health—or, at least, part of it.*

Applying a CGM is initially harrowing for trypanophobes like me (those of us who don't adore needles). You must puncture the skin with a miniscule sticker. Once applied, a small filament attached to the sensor remains under the skin, allowing the device to measure glucose levels via interstitial fluid. The sensor then bounces its data to a phone app, which displays your blood glucose levels moment to moment. After three rounds of deep belly breathing, I snapped mine into place without the slightest wince of pain.

You would never drive a car without a functioning dashboard. When the oil or tire pressure light is illuminated, you might blow it off for a day or two. But if it remained lit, you would likely address it. A CGM is a dashboard into your own physiological vehicle, one that you cannot replace with another lease.

As I stared into the app, to my shock, my "check engine" light was on. My fasting blood glucose was hovering around 125 mg/dL with post-prandial (after meal) spikes of 200 and north. This blood sugar level put me squarely into the category of prediabetes and on the cusp of full-fledged diabetes.

Even worse, I understood that while blood glucose is a decent metric and relatively easy to measure, it is downstream from insulin, the peptide hormone tasked with ushering glucose out of the bloodstream. Your pancreas can keep blood sugar within the normal range by pumping out excess insulin. But that stage was already in my rearview mirror. My elevated glucose levels were indicative of insulin resistance. Despite the arduous work of my dutiful pancreas, my cells had become resistant to its product. As I would discover, the excess of any molecule in the body produces a resistance to itself. I knew this by analogy with Merlot and espresso. Apparently, it was also true with insulin.

* Originally developed for diabetics, CGMs have now become available to the general public. At this juncture, they are not inexpensive, but as demand rises and insurers come around to the wisdom that it's cheaper to prevent diabetes than to treat it, CGMs should become more democratically available.

Insulin resistance creates a vicious cycle as the body produces more and more insulin to compensate. This leads to a parallel condition known as hyperinsulinemia.

Metabolic dysfunction often reflected by glucose imbalance, insulin resistance, and hyperinsulinemia is directly associated with all the FUCKs: cardiovascular disease, cancer, Alzheimer's, and diabetes.

Here's the curious thing: I thought I was pretty healthy. I exercised regularly. I shopped at Whole Foods. My annual visits with my primary care physician, when I didn't cancel them, came and went without incident. I was a productive member of society, raising children and paying my taxes. For God's sake, I ran a wellness company!

But, in reality, I wasn't at all healthy. I was living the nightmare—and not in its early chapters. I wasn't yet being chased through the woods, but the chainsaw was revving in some creepy, cob-webbed cabin.

Like 93 percent of Americans, I had metabolic dysfunction. And, because the symptoms seemed so humdrum and common, I wasn't aware of the slippery slope I was sliding down.

But the early warning signs that I was FUCK'd were glaringly obvious, as soon as I knew where to look.

I had the aforementioned brain fog and chronic fatigue, a direct result of my mitochondria's impaired ability to produce energy. I was fidgety and irritable and had a hard time focusing. Reading a book, or even a nutrition label, seemed utterly implausible, given my knee-jerk reflex to needlessly yet constantly check my phone. I was prone to mood swings and excessively triggered by politics and current affairs. I had grown a patently unattractive brown skin tag in my right armpit, another presentation of insulin resistance. My waist-to-hip ratio was north of 1. It should hover around 0.8.

I had "dad bod"—fat deposition around my abdomen, a good indication of visceral and ectopic fat. This type of fat around and in your organs can be both a cause and an effect of insulin resistance. I had early onset man boobs—and not just A-cups. Later, I was told I had a leak in my gut. I didn't initially know what that meant, but it didn't sound great.

Can you relate to any of this?

Like so many modern humans, I had gotten soft both in the middle and in the mind. Creature comforts had dulled my sharper edges and, as I will explain, were leveraging my biology against me. I had gotten wickedly out of balance, and something needed to change. I needed to unFUCK myself.

The following chapters distill my journey to realign myself with my own biology and reclaim my health and vitality. They are a confection of all the knowledge that I have gleaned from doctors, thinkers, and wellness practitioners as well as a ton of "mesearch." As I will describe, my exploration included both the metaphysical and the physical, the strategic and the tactical. Initially, and surprisingly, I didn't find the clues of health's origins in PubMed but rather scrawled in ancient texts. Before I could "be" healthy, I had to understand what health was.

The good news—the gospel—is that when we are realigned with our adaptive design through the protocols I outline, it is astounding how quickly the body responds and begins to heal. Our fates are not fixed. We have tremendous agency.

I want to be 118 in that cabin. And I want you to be there too. Well, preferably, in your own cabin.

Some History

Before going forward, let me take you briefly backward to provide the full arc of my health dramedy. Consider this my bio-psycho-social intake form. I suggest you also find the opportunity to fill one out.

Much of our physiological and psychological state have their roots in our past. Our present is shaped through patterns that are woven into the lattice work of our lives. Thus, a significant part of my healing journey included taking an honest inventory of my childhood.

I'll spare you a lengthy biography for another time. But I will provide a somewhat frosted window into my peripatetic upbringing. My parents moved me 11 times before I was seven. My itinerant youth was a thicket of both wonder and despair.

As a young babe, I was perambulated through the lush landscapes of the Lake District of Northern England. My memory is about as foggy as the damp, dewy mornings, but I do recall the endless bounty of fresh berries of every variety. As I got older, my mother and I would mosey out on my pony, who I dubbed "Maybe." I always had a non-committal streak in matters of naming, as my daughters can attest.

We would fill buckets until they were brimming with luscious and fecund mulberries, blueberries, and blackberries and shuttle them back to the kitchen where Mrs. Pat was baking fresh bread. She would supervise the crushing of the berries. She'd then simmer them, letting me add the sugar, until the pectin released and the mixture thickened into a spreadable jam. The comfort of fresh bread and homemade jam is what I remember best of Northern England.

When I was three, my family moved to Spain. I attended preschool in the picturesque town of Santiago de Compostela, where I wore one shoe that had an additional block of cork affixed to the bottom. This ham-fisted feature was designed to address my hip dysplasia but evidently not to win me many friends.

Further, my preternaturally chubby cheeks were the target of the wrinkly, bony fingers of street-strolling gray-haired Spanish abuelas. On more than one occasion, a dotty old bat on the sidewalk would unilaterally lunge at me to pinch my fleshy face, only to be met with a block of cork swung swiftly into her shin.

In 1974, my parents transplanted me to Rio de Janeiro, Brazil, and enrolled me in kindergarten at the American School. There was a mix of students, mostly Brazilian and a smattering of foreign nationals from the United States, Britain, and other parts of Europe. English was predominant in the classroom. But, on the playground, the linguistic currency was Portuguese, specifically Carioca, the slangy dialect native to Rio.

My absorbent brain sponged up the language like Bounty. The transition from Galician Spanish to Portuguese was simpler for the nonconceptual child brain. I was trading in sounds, language as music, not as vocabulary lessons. And, of course, I was heaved into fluency by a force greater than anything cognitive: the innate instinct to belong.

We all have our childhood traumas—both big *T* trauma-inducing events and little *t* chronic-trauma-inducing ones. We too often carry these adverse childhood experiences around like rucksacks into adulthood. In my interview with trauma specialist Peter Levine, he called these burdens "the tyranny of the past." If I could reduce my childhood suffering into a singular *tyrannical* ordeal, it would be this one:

It was recess.

Kids were peppered across the playground, playing and hollering. The yard outside the main school building was sloped at one end. And it was a favorite pastime to sprint along the flat section of the lawn and then jump onto your bum and slide down the grade. Due to this repetitive activity, the grass had given way to dirt halfway down the incline, forming an earthen landing strip of sorts.

This was a ritual that I conscientiously avoided. My body wasn't engineered for such nimble maneuvers. I was chubby. My paunch belly hung over my jeans. The denim between my chafing thighs had been rendered smooth and threadbare.

I lingered on the sidelines, listening to the school bully, Bobbito, direct traffic down the slope. The soundscape was frenzied and chaotic. What possessed me I don't remember, but a sudden surge of self-confidence propelled me into line, and I poised myself the best I could.

My turn. Big inhale. Go. I scampered toward the slope and flung myself awkwardly like a baby robin's first flight out of the nest. It wasn't the smoothest landing, and certainly no distance records were set, but I did it. I made it down the slope. A couple barks of "Americano" were my reward.

Now, more sure of myself, I trudged back up the hill back into the queue. I cinched my belt a notch, tugged on my polo. This time my approach had more verve. I launched up, landed on my butt—and heard the sound.

It was a ripping noise that momentarily transcended all other components of existence. I had torn my jeans straight down the crack of my ass. What's more, my tighty-whities, now visually available to the yard, had been stained by the dirt path.

This momentous misfortune sent Bobbito into paroxysms of rapturous laughter and joy as he belted out, "The American shat his pants." The refrain was repeated again and again. "The American shat his pants. The American shat his pants." A catchy tune it must have been as it echoed across the yard. I stood at the bottom of the hill, naked, nowhere to hide, eyes welled, lip bit with nothing but self-hatred and embarrassment.

Fight, flight, freeze, or, in this case, find the angle from which the least amount of people can see your stained underwear, then shuffle back to the classrooms. Finally, off the Serengeti and back in the relative safety of the school, I found my backpack and slung it awkwardly behind me in an attempt to camouflage my accident. I limped into the nurse's office purporting an awful headache—one that apparently must have caused the nurse to think I shat my pants.

"I have to go home," I told her. "I must go home!" My mother was summoned and dutifully arrived. I made my brisk walk of shame back across the yard, clumsily as if I was in a three-legged race with myself. One last lingering coda of the "the American shat his pants" faded into the distance.

This was the mythology of my youth, the polar opposite of the hero's journey, replete with all its classic shadow archetypes: the bully, the nurse, the tender mother, the ego, the shame, the self-loathing.

The incessant bouncing from country to country that I bore as a child had its benefits. I was immersed in various cultures and enjoyed their trappings. The left hemisphere of my brain, the locus of language, was a flourishing garden. But every year, my social connections were erased and I was forced to begin again . . . wiggling my way like a fat worm into preexisting cliques of friends in a new school in a new country in a new dialect.

And this struggle became the story of my life: the incessant need to fit in, to be liked, to assimilate, to seek the approval of others, to base my identity on what other people thought of me.

It was this proclivity that led me to get into a taxicab 35 years later with my three daughters, recognize that the driver was Jamaican, and subconsciously muster a thick Rastafarian accent, "Take me uptown, mon!" as if a giant dreadlock had sprung from my head. My girls looked at me, horrified and embarrassed, as the cabbie eyed my undeniable whiteness with confusion and pity.

This phenomenon presses on. If you listen to my podcast, you'll quickly notice the accents I spontaneously adopt with various guests: a southern drawl with Matthew McConaughey, a cockney brogue with Russell Brand, a thundering Viking-like Dutch bur with Wim Hof, a foray into Hinglish with Deepak Chopra.

This penchant is bottom-up. It emerges from below the crust of consciousness. It has become a biological imperative—an involuntary adaptive dance that I subconsciously implement for the purpose of connection.

The social scientist Brené Brown makes an astute distinction between fitting in and belonging. *Fitting in* is changing who you are in order to be accepted. *Belonging* is being accepted while never compromising your authentic self. Of course, a five-year-old isn't equipped to make this delineation. The renowned trauma expert Gabor Maté contends that people, especially children, will always sacrifice authenticity for attachment. In other words, the need for connection trumps our yearning to be our true selves.

I share this background because, like so many people, I *became* my personal folklore. My identity was anchored in the stories I told myself about myself. My favorite refrains were:

I'm not enough.

I lost the genetic lottery.

I had the thrifty gene, useful in a famine but patently not on the playground.

I just *had* bad metabolism.

Being fat was just who I was.

I'll never belong.

I clutched onto this version of myself as if it were a security blanket, or, more appropriately, an insecurity blanket. I was the heavy kid who would do anything to be liked. Even in my more slender adolescence, and still persisting today, when I look in the mirror, I see a sweaty, chubby kid whose pitiful fate was written in the stars.

This narrative followed me until adult life. The conditions it engendered weren't completely debilitating and, in a way, that made it worse. If I had had a "critical" condition, then perhaps I would have been forced to deal with it. Instead, I was limping through life, quite literally. At 41, I had a total left hip replacement. By 49, I was a 206-pound, exhausted, inflamed, chronically sick diabetic with a leaky gut.

In other words, I was an average American.

CHAPTER 3

THE JOURNEY BEGINS

Science is not only compatible with spirituality; it is a profound source of spirituality.
— Carl Sagan

My healing journey didn't initially begin with the adoption of any specific set of protocols but rather with a road trip. My awakening wasn't even initially physiological. It was more metaphysical than physical.

That sounds awfully pompous. I was hardly raking pea gravel in a saffron robe. However, as I will describe, I got a glimpse into the understory of well-being. I began to understand human physiology within the greater context of nature, and, by extension, how my own organism functioned as nature. The key to health, I realized, was leveraging nature's operating system adaptively. It took me years to figure it out, but over time, I developed a philosophy that eventually informed the tactics of Good Stress.

Candidly, I wasn't even actively seeking healing in 2018. But, as I have described, I desperately needed it. I suppose "when the student is ready, the teacher will appear."

That summer, I convinced my eldest daughter, Phoebe, to take a road trip up the California coast to visit colleges. Candidly, the entire trip was a bit premature, flimsily camouflaging my need to cling to my waning paternal utility. Nevertheless, Phoebe, in a moment of pity, agreed to the excursion, assuming we'd be cashing in Hilton Honors points.

She was astonished to witness me pulling up the driveway in an army-green camper van that I had rented for the trip. She turned quickly pale, realizing there'd be no ice machines and hotel room Nespresso. She and her dear old dad were going to snake up the golden coastline in a well-appointed Winnebago, roasting vegan marshmallows, crashing at campsites, and sleeping snugly in the cargo bay.

It was exciting—for about 20 minutes. As the exhilaration lost its luster, we started fidgeting with the radio. What were we going to listen to for the next 40-some hours?

A month prior to this trip, I had made the acquaintance of Mark Watts. Mark is the son of Alan Watts, the brilliant British philosopher. I was vaguely familiar with Watts at this juncture, mostly by account of YouTube, which features all sorts of Watts snippets remixed to ambient beats. Mark is the more than capable steward of his father's estate and library. As a teenager, Mark traveled with his father and oversaw the recording of countless lectures on an old reel-to-reel tape machine. Mark had archived these fossil records as well as the many discourses his father delivered on San Francisco–based KQED radio.

In the 1950s and 1960s, Alan Watts was central to introducing the West to Eastern religions, including Taoism, Hinduism, Buddhism, and Zen. He appealed to both the beatniks and the hippies and consorted with the likes of Aldous Huxley and Krishnamurti. Watts was an infamous Epicurean and self-admitted rascal, prone to excessive pleasures of the flesh. However, he was unrivaled in his oratorical clarity and humor. Sadly, Watts passed on much too early, likely due to vice, in 1973 at the age of 58.

Mark was generous enough to license a large swath of his father's catalog to Commune, my media company. It was my job to curate the bits and pieces of these lectures that would eventually inform a Commune online course on Eastern religions. Hence, I downloaded hundreds of hours of discourses onto my phone prior to embarking with Phoebe.

"How about we listen to Alan Watts?" I suggested as we inched along the 101. Phoebe did not demur.

We began listening to "Man & Nature" from a collection titled the *Tao of Philosophy*. As the track began, the analog audio popped and crackled, lending an immediate authenticity to the soundtrack. Watts then started in with his inimitable BBC transatlantic accent, "In my talk last night, I was discussing the disparity between the way in which most human beings experience their own existence and the way man's being and nature is described in the sciences."

We were hooked.

From UCLA to UC Santa Barbara, from UC Santa Cruz to UC Berkeley, from UC Davis to UC Riverside, we listened exclusively to Watts. My zeal for his lectures continued after my return to the City of Angels and reached its apogee after I contracted COVID in March 2020. Watts, along with the spiritual teacher Mooji, were my buoys as I swam against the currents of the virus. I spent hours melting in the sauna, meditating to their oratory.

It is ironic that a man so committed to potato vodka spurred me on my quest for well-being. Of course, it wasn't his personal foibles that propelled me. It was his insight into the nature of being.

I continued to listen endlessly to Watts unpack Eastern mysticism as I meandered the hiking trails of the Santa Monica Mountains. I had also licensed a significant portion of lecture content from the great American spiritualist Ram Dass from Raghu Markus at the Be Here Now Network. Ram Dass, formerly Richard Alpert, also became my regular walking companion. Additionally, I interviewed Deepak Chopra a number of times, as well as Davidji, Yung Pueblo, Sharon Salzberg, and others about Eastern philosophy.

As I dove deep into the metaphysical, I also began trying to understand why I was physically so compromised. This inquiry led me to interview every doctor who would speak to me, from Mark Hyman to Sara Gottfried, from Robert Lustig to Andrew Huberman, from Casey Means to Benjamin Bikman, and hundreds of others.

In a moment of satori, these two separate inquests converged. The tenets of Eastern mysticism were everywhere to be found in my body. The human organism was, as the Buddha posited, impermanent and interdependent with its environment, spontaneously arising at all times in relation to everything else.

Like nature more broadly, the body has a Tao—a fundamental intelligence that brings countervailing processes and molecules into balance and equilibrium. To be healthy, I needed to understand the opposing forces within my organism and cultivate a "middle way." I needed to bring imbalances back into balance.

Of course, this was not a completely new insight. This concept is central to various forms of Eastern medicine. In Ayurveda, India's 3,000-year-old natural system of medicine, perfect health is defined as a balance between body, mind, spirit, and social well-being. An Ayurvedic doctor seeks to create a state of equilibrium between a patient's *doshas* (the fundamental physiological governing principles of the body), *agni* (metabolic and digestive processes), and *dhatu* (principles that uphold the formation of body tissues).

In traditional Chinese medicine, practitioners seek to achieve balance between the internal body organs and the external elements of earth, fire, water, wood, and metal. There is a focus on harmonizing dryness and dampness and clearing meridians to enable the flow of qi (life force) through the body.

These traditions, however, developed without the benefit of the tools of modern medicine that allow us to probe human physiology at its empirical roots. We can now study how the metaphysical is patterned in the physical through an arsenal of machines and wearables, from fMRIs to Oura rings.

Across my journey, I began to slowly assemble a philosophy for well-being that I call the Tao of Health. This philosophy merged a Western empirical understanding of physiology with the principles of Eastern thought. Its four principles—impermanence, interdependence, agency, and balance—would become the root system for Good Stress.

CHAPTER 4

THE TAO OF HEALTH PRINCIPLE #1

Impermanence (You Are a Flame)

This existence of ours is as transient as autumn clouds. To watch the birth and death of beings is like looking at the movements of a dance. A lifetime is like a flash of lightning in the sky, rushing by like a torrent down a steep mountain.

— Buddha

Before I could change my body, I needed to wake up to the notion that change was actually possible. My entire life had been riddled by ideas like "I just have a slow metabolism"—as if a metabolism was a fixed thing that one might possess, like an ugly sweater hanging haplessly in a closet. I have many such sweaters.

More recently, in an interview I conducted with Dr. William Li, I learned that, contrary to popular myth, one's core metabolism barely degrades at all between ages 20 and 60. And, from a genetic perspective, there is very little variability in metabolic rate from one person to the next. This news violated my long-held fealty to genetic determinism.

At the beginning of my journey, however, in order to feel a sense of agency over my own health, I had to learn a lesson as old as the Buddha: there is no stable, reliable self. Each one of us is a fluctuating process. We are impermanent.

Let me illuminate this revelation by analogy with a BIC lighter. You've likely toyed with one in your party days. Well, you have more in common with this plastic flame-thrower than you might initially think.

When you run your thumb across the flint wheel, you generate a spark. This ignition mechanism activates a chemical reaction between the fuel source and oxygen in the air. This reaction results in combustion. An orange flame flares atop a hotter blue base. The energy substrate being leveraged is butane, the chemical formula of which is C_4H_{10}.

The flame flickers but largely maintains the same form. As you stare at it, however, you know innately that all the molecules involved in this phenomenon are simply moving on. It's an ongoing reaction producing heat, water vapor, and carbon dioxide.

Curiously, you also use hydrocarbon fuel substrates in the form of carbohydrates and fats in combination with oxygen to make energy. Carbs and fats are long-chain carbon molecules flanked by hydrogen and oxygen. And you generate the same by-products as the BIC lighter: heat, water, and carbon dioxide.

Like a flame, you are recognizable by your form. And, like a flame, every molecule that "informs" your morphology moves on moment by moment. Your physiology is completely impermanent.

Let me paint it another way. Have you ever visited a waterfall and found it so delightful that you visited it again and again? How did you recognize it from one visit to another? Of course, you recognized it by its form—the height and width of its brink, the turbidity of the water, the rocks jutting up from its plunge. But, at the same time, you intuitively knew that all the molecules of water that you saw yesterday had moved on downstream.

This description can be faithfully applied to what you call "yourself." Your best friend recognizes you day-to-day by your form: your hair, eye, and skin color.

But just as the molecules of H_2O have gone downriver, everything that makes you up has moved on. You are like a lighter's flame, a series of trillions upon trillions of chemical reactions—pilfering oxygen, creating and expending energy, and by-producing carbon dioxide and water.

There are, last I counted, approximately 70 trillion cells in the human body, and 39 trillion of them are prokaryotic single-celled nonhuman organisms—mostly bacteria snuggled in the colon. They coexist somewhat acrimoniously with fungi, archaea, and 380 trillion viruses (viruses are not cells). The lifespan of these bacteria varies between 4 minutes and 24 hours. You've turned over trillions of cells since you started reading this chapter. There is nothing stable or fixed about being human. You're an ever-changing process.

Let me further underscore our impermanence by taking a gander at the lifespan of human cells:[1]

- Neutrophil cells: 2 days
- Cells lining the gut epithelium: 5 days
- White blood cells: 13 days
- Red blood cells: 120 days
- Liver cells: 10 to 16 months
- Pancreas cells: 1 year
- Hematopoietic stem cells: 5 years
- Skeletal muscle cells: 15.1 years
- Intestinal cells (excluding lining): 15.9 years
- Heart muscle cells: 40 years

However, simply grokking the ephemerality of cells is to say nothing about the impermanence of oxygen picking up electrons in the mitochondria, glycolysis breaking down glucose into pyruvate, muscles burning ATP, antioxidants neutering free radicals, immune cells gobbling up bacteria, electromagnetic signals zipping across synapses, and on and on and on. There are 37 billion billion (that's not a typo, it's 37 *billion billion*) chemical reactions occurring in your body every second.

If you think you're the same person now that started reading this book, then let me disabuse you of this notion. Everything that makes you up has flowed downstream. The myth that "you can't change" is apocryphal. All you do is change.

Do you find this perplexing? I do, because I don't feel impermanent. I feel like a stable thing, anchored to my sense of self through a feeling of physical continuity. I get out of the shower, study myself vainly and meticulously in the mirror as I suck in my gut and flex my pectorals. I look, more or less, the same day-to-day.

However, a mere flip through a photo album is enough to demonstrate that nothing about my physical organism endures. Am I the cherubic baby huddled in my adoring mother's arms; the disheveled, stoned college student; or the distinguished denizen of middle age that types this paragraph?

Of course, I am none of these things. I am a process, spontaneously emerging moment to moment in relationship to my environment. Even my DNA, the fixed nucleotide sequences that form the foundation of my genes, expresses itself differently in connection to the inputs of my ecosystem.

Once I accepted the transience of my body, it was easy to surrender to the notion that, from a physiological perspective, there was nothing remotely stable or permanent to my being. My body is a constantly evolving process distinguishable day-to-day by its form.

This "awakening" to my physical impermanence was reflective of the Buddha's realization of Anatman, the non-self. Spiritually, this transformation is crucial to the Buddhist notion of liberation. But it also has profound implications physiologically.

Why is the concept of impermanence important to health? Well, if I am "a process" and not a fixed product, then so are diseases. They are processes too, evolving moment to moment. They exist along a spectrum. Moment to moment, I am either healing—moving toward wholeness—or ailing and moving toward disconnection and illness.

As I awoke to my body's transience, I began to ask myself this essential question: If I am a flame, then how brightly will I shine?

We've all sat around a raging fire where the flames are jumping and flashing. And we've likely all witnessed a candle's flame on the edge of extinguishment. The difference between the two is obvious.

From a technical perspective, energy in the human body is made by the mitochondria, tiny little organelles in our cells. These cellular power plants were the result of a blind date between a bacterium and an archaea cell 2 billion years ago. This ancient tryst led to aerobic respiration—the ability to make energy with oxygen—and spurred on complex multicellular life. How efficiently your mitochondria utilize carbohydrates, fats, and oxygen determines how brightly your flame shines.

When I took an honest look at myself in 2019, I realized my glow was barely a flicker.

Of course, there are many ways that we differ from a BIC lighter. A lighter can't procreate. You can bang two BIC lighters against each other all day. Like Barbie and Ken, they won't produce another one. A lighter won't heal itself when the parts break. And it dies when it runs out of fuel.

You and I will die too. But, during this wild and wondrous life, the power to shine, to brighten our flame, is largely in our control. Like adding more wood or pumping a bellows, we can stoke our inner fire.

Key Learnings:

1. Our organism is not fixed. It is constantly in flux.
2. Our organism is a process that moves along a spectrum from well to unwell, from ease to disease.
3. By extension, disease is also a process.
4. We can be moving along this spectrum toward wholeness—the process of healing—or toward disease—the process of ailing.

CHAPTER 5

THE TAO OF HEALTH PRINCIPLE #2

Interdependence (Indra's Net)

Imagine a multidimensional spider's web in the early morning covered with dew drops. And every dew drop contains the reflection of all the other dew drops. And, in each reflected dew drop, the reflections of all the other dew drops in that reflection, and so on ad infinitum. That is the Buddhist conception of the universe in an image.

— Alan Watts

Most of the time, we humans trudge through life feeling separate from the world around us. We identify as a locus of consciousness situated somewhere behind the eyes, locked up in an increasingly saggy bag of skin, divorced from the "external" world. We feel like an individual.

However, this sensation of being a separate self is in conflict not only with the study of human physiology but also with direct experience. For example, on even pavement, you walk at a pace of about three miles per hour. But, of course, you walk slower up a steep grade and even slower than that in sand and even slower than that in water. The behavior of walking is inseparable from the topography upon which you walk.

The Alan Watts lecture titled "A Coincidence of Opposites" was one that looped in my AirPods like a Mobius strip. One of its primary teachings was this concept:

You cannot define your function and behavior as separate from the function and behavior of your environment.

One morning in Topanga, I sat in the sauna sweating buckets with Dr. Mark Hyman. As I spooned water onto the hot rocks, Mark introduced me to a new word: *exposome.*

Exposome is the term for the sum total of all the exposures in our lifetime, from the womb to the tomb. These exposures include the food we eat, environmental toxins and heavy metals, the air we breathe, the water we drink, and even our thoughts and emotions.

While your genes play some role, for the most part, they are not the main determinant of our health. According to Mark, what matters more is this exposome—the environment to which your genes are exposed. In fact, over 90 percent of chronic disease is determined by the food you eat, stress, thoughts, relationships, feelings, and toxins, all washing over your genes.

The study of how gene expression modifies in relationship to behavior and the environment is called epigenetics. I will return to this concept in a moment.

The cogitations of Watts and Hyman were different spokes converging toward a central hub. To be alive is to be in relationship. Again, you cannot define the function and behavior of your organism outside of the function and behavior of your environment. You and your ecosystem are mutually interdependent. They arise simultaneously.

Let me illustrate this point through playing an imaginary nefarious trick on you.

I furtively sneak up behind you and scream bloody murder in your ear. What happens to you?

My unexpected piercing scream startles you, hijacks your amygdala, and sends an instantaneous signal down your HPA axis to release cortisol, which sends glucose to your muscles and increases heart and respiratory rate. An arbitrary noise from the outside world is an endocrine disruptor.

Even more perplexing, this sound is just a wave of amplitudes and frequencies in the putative external world. It's not until these vibrations are converted to electric impulses delivered down the auditory nerve to your brain that my scream becomes a sound. And then your mind gets in the act and layers a valence and salience on top of it. A soundless invisible waveform is responsible for your adrenal gland producing a stress hormone from cholesterol. In this scenario, intention and energy combine to become matter.

That's astounding.

Further, sound is purely a neurological phenomenon. In this sense, the external world is internal. The inside of your brain sounds like the outside. And you move, live, and cook dinner in the external world. Or perhaps there is no difference. You are an environment-organism. An environism. An organment.

Let me further cement this notion of interdependence with the world by discussing the contents of my colon. I'm sure that's what you're here for.

Across three daughters, I changed a lot of diapers. Okay, Schuyler changed more. Still our household was not some portrait of medieval patriarchy. I handled my fair share of shitty nappies over the years. That said, I don't love handling poop, at least not as much as Dr. Mary Pardee does. Mary is a poop specialist. Technically, she's a gastroenterologist, but most of our conversations float atop what is emitted from my anus.

In a devious way, interviewing all these doctors was a method of getting free expert medical advice. When I podded with Mary, she suggested that I get a poop test, more properly known as a microbiome analysis. This test examines the microorganisms, particularly bacteria, present in my colon.

My labs had revealed a high level of C-reactive protein, a biomarker indicative of systemic inflammation. It was possible that this inflammation was due to a leaky gut, clinically known as intestinal permeability.

I was interested in what my poop exam might reveal about my health. I was less interested in the sample collection aspect of the test. There's a lot of indignity in being healthy, and the self-administration of the pooper scooper hovers near the top of that list. Despite my squeamishness, in a moment of great courage, I harvested my poop in a strainer, clumsily stuffed it in the specimen cup, and shipped it off to a lab. I do hope the technicians in a poop lab receive a proper wage for the duty of handling doody.

A week later, I received the results. Indeed, I had dysbiosis. A suspect diet with too much sugar, chronic stress, and wicked insomnia had conspired to massacre my good gut bugs and help the damaging ones to proliferate. Further, there was evidence to suggest that the tight junctions in my gut lining had eroded. I'll explain why these conditions are so detrimental to health in a moment. But, before I do, I must share with you my astounding realization.

These nonhuman bacterial cells that I had collected in utero and from breast milk, foodstuffs, hugs, kisses, and toilet handles were a major determinant of my health. And, in turn, I was essential to theirs. We were mutually interdependent.

There may be no better representation of the body as transient and inseparable from its environment than the vast colony of bugs nestling primarily in the gut. The human organism consists of about 70 trillion cells. Approximately 30 trillion of these cells are human and contain your DNA;[1] 99.9 percent of my genetic blueprint matches yours, no matter who you are.[2] And, for this, I apologize.

The balance of the cells in your body are prokaryotes in the form of bacteria, archaea, and fungi. These single-celled organisms make up your microbiota. They reside in your mouth, on your skin, and, increasingly, they have been discovered in every organ system—but, predominantly, they can be found partying down in the anaerobic den of iniquity known as your colon. On a good day, there are upward of 1,000 species of bacteria embedded in the walls of your colon's mucosal epithelium, and each of them has its own proper genome.

There are 3.3 million nonredundant genes in your gut microbiome alone[3] as compared to the measly 22,300 genes in your own DNA.[4] Put together, here is some rough math: your genetic makeup is 150 times more bacterial than human.

These bacteria have input into the functionality of nearly every system of your body. Increasingly, it appears as if human life—including human health and disease—is not centered exclusively around the human cell.

The dominant gut microbial phyla are *Firmicutes* and *Bacteroidetes*. Bacteria propagate primarily through binary fission. In essence, they reach a predetermined girth and split in two. If Americans reproduced in the same manner, it would undoubtedly solve the problem of low birth rates.

Your gut bacteria are transitory buggers with a lifespan of between 4 minutes and 24 hours. In this sense, during the time it took me to fly from Los Angeles to Paris to visit my daughter, more than 50 percent of what makes up my organism had come and gone. I was not the same person when I landed at Charles de Gaulle as I was when I departed LAX.

While you might own the apartment complex of your organism, your bug tenants have great influence over how well the building functions. If you are a responsive landlord, they pay their rent. If you're not, your organism can quickly become a bordello.

Much of the food you consume gets digested and leveraged by your body. What does not get digested and absorbed in the small intestine flows into the colon and becomes sustenance for your gut bugs. Health-conferring bacteria thrive when they are fed well and, in turn, are upstanding members of the community. I will discuss their preferred diet in detail later. But when friendly bacteria like *Lactobacillus* get prebiotic fiber, they will produce postbiotics, the most famous of which is butyrate, a short-chain fatty acid. Butyrate is a superhero molecule that provides energy for colon cells, regulates inflammation, increases insulin sensitivity, influences gene expression, and even prevents cancer.

When gut bacteria are fed poorly, the affable ones move out and the rapscallion bugs like *Clostridium difficile*, *Helicobacter pylori*, and *Escherichia coli* move in. You may know these characters by their street names: *C. diff*, *H. pylori*, and *E. coli*. These bacteria can cause symptoms ranging from diarrhea to life-threatening inflammation of the colon.

Sadly, the modern Western diet is laden with compounds that create bacterial imbalances in the gut. This condition is known as dysbiosis. *Dysbiosis* refers to an imbalance in the microbiota, involving a reduction in the diversity of bacteria, an overgrowth of potentially harmful bacteria, or a decrease in beneficial bacteria. It is often associated with disorders like inflammatory bowel disease (IBD), irritable bowel syndrome (IBS), small intestinal bacterial overgrowth (SIBO), obesity, and even mental health disorders. Indeed, your gut and your brain are connected.

There's a Leak in My Gut

This feels like a very intimate share, but my gut was as leaky as a rusty old pipe. The contents of the colon are separated from the bloodstream by the epithelial wall. It is literally one cell thick. It reminds me of the wall in my college dorm room. I could hear everything that happened next door. I may write that lurid novel for a different section of the bookstore.

The integrity of this wall is held together by tight junctions between the epithelial cells. When dysregulation of the gut microbiome occurs, these tight junctions can erode, and endotoxins can pass into the bloodstream.

Intestinal permeability, gruesomely nicknamed "leaky gut," is a condition where the lining of the small intestine becomes damaged. This can cause undigested food particles, toxic waste products, and endotoxins to "leak" through the intestines and into the bloodstream.

Endotoxins are harmful compounds that are released when a bacterial cell disintegrates. Lipopolysaccharides are notorious endotoxins. They are part of bacterial cell membranes that decompose and then enter the bloodstream. LPS (dubbed "little pieces of shit" by the ever-comedic Dr. Stephen Gundry) have substantial impacts on human health, primarily through interactions with the immune system.

In a bacterially balanced gut, the intestinal lining is selectively permeable, which means it controls what gets absorbed into the bloodstream from the digestive tract. It allows nutrients to pass through while preventing harmful substances from entering. In healthy intestines, tight junctions exist between the cells (enterocytes) lining the intestinal wall, allowing this selectivity. However, when these tight junctions become "loose" or the integrity of the intestinal lining is compromised, increased intestinal permeability or leaky gut can occur.

In my 30s and 40s, I had engaged in just about every behavior that would cause a gut to leak. I indulged in bagels, cookies, and India Pale Ales. Mmmm. . . beer. Post-tennis, I'd pop nonsteroidal anti-inflammatory drugs (NSAIDs) such as Advil like popcorn. Then, after abusing my gastrointestinal tract, I'd wonder why it felt like an acid pit. In retaliation, I would take proton pump inhibitors (PPIs) like Prilosec and Nexium. And, the icing—chocolate, please—on the cake was chronic stress.

All these behaviors, in conjunction with the consumption of broad-spectrum antibiotics, environmental toxins, and herbicide-ridden foods, combined to create a caustic exposome for my gut. And I suffered the consequences. The Big MACs had turned my biology against me.

The degradation of my gut lining led to a chronic activation of my immune system as toxins that should have been destined for the toilet bowl entered my bloodstream instead. My immune system was just doing what it was supposed to do: send white blood cells to the site of the insult. This is called inflammation. Inflammation is a brilliant adaptive response when you twist your ankle. Like modern medicine, inflammation is a potent tool for acute injury. Like stress, inflammation is maladaptive when it is chronic.

The systemic chronic inflammation due to my leaky gut was contributing to my metabolic dysfunction. Indeed, chronic inflammation sits upstream from nearly every modern disease, including mental health disorders, autoimmune diseases, and cardiovascular diseases.

Despite the poor state of my gastrointestinal affairs, a light bulb appeared brightly above my head. As I alternated between Watts and Hyman, a bolt of electricity passed through the filament of my brain and lit it up.

My organism is a process. This process exists on a spectrum between well and unwell. The status of this process is regulated by its exposome. This notion is, at its core, empowering because I have significant agency over my exposome.

If indeed "all disease begins in the gut" as Hippocrates, the father of modern medicine, proclaimed, then I had a choice. I could cultivate an environment for my gut bugs to thrive. I could feed them delicious fiber, phytonutrients, and polyphenols, thus nurturing a friendly intestinal population.

In turn, they would produce the metabolites that improve insulin sensitivity, regulate mood, maintain gut barrier integrity, and foster a more balanced immune system. In this miraculous interdependent universe, humans have co-evolved with bacteria to look after each other.

Oddly, the study of the microbiota inspired a moment of satori. The microscope widens the aperture of the macroscope. Humans don't exist as separate disjointed selves—living in a separate external universe, separate from nature and from each other. On the contrary, we live within a holobiont of interconnected and mutually reliant organisms and genomics.

Looking deep into my physical bowels unveiled a metaphysical concept. Again, the medical and mystical converged.

Eastern mysticism and modern biology share a common essence: the awareness of the unity and mutual interrelation of all things and events. The properties of any object or system can only be understood as a relationship between things. This is true at every level—from the behavior of atoms to the function of organs to the conduct of humans.

This concept is consilient across a plethora of spiritual traditions. *Pratītyasamutpāda*, or dependent origination, is the Buddhist doctrine of interdependence. Mutual arising is also a signature of Taoism. In Japanese, this concept is known as *Jijimuge*, the interpenetration of all phenomena. Between every thing or event (ji) and every other thing or event there is no (mu) barrier (ge). *Ubuntu* is an African concept that is often translated as "I am because we are." In Xhosa, the term is used philosophically to mean "the belief in a universal bond of sharing that connects all humanity."

I began to understand that my organism was woven into the fabric of an infinite web, a connected and inseparable part of a cosmic whole. I was a diamond reflecting the total energy of the universe. I was living within Indra's net.

Key Learnings:

1. We are interdependent beings. Our health is inextricably connected to the health of everything around us.
2. You cannot separate the function and behavior of an organism from the function and behavior of its environment.

CHAPTER 6

THE TAO OF HEALTH PRINCIPLE #3

The Age of Agency (You Have Less Genes Than a Grape)

The power to define your health destiny lies much more in your hands than it does in your genes.

— DR. DAVID KATZ

My emerging understanding of my organism as impermanent and interdependent with its environment started to upend my long-held beliefs that my health destiny was predetermined.

How many of us have attributed an autoimmune disease or weight problem or chronic condition to genetics? I did. For years, I said both aloud and to myself, "I just have slow metabolism. It's in my genes. I was born that way, and there's very little I can do about it."

But the more doctors I spoke with, the less stock I began to put in the notion that my fate was predestined by fixed underlying mechanisms. No one was more influential in this respect than Dr. Zach Bush.

On a cool night in 2020, I sat with Zach on the patio in Topanga. We were winding down after a fundraiser for Farmer's Footprint, a nonprofit focused on regenerative agriculture. An abandoned bowl of fruit salad lingered on the table. I mindlessly pushed a green grape around the bowl with a bamboo fork.

"More genes than you," Zach quipped offhandedly.

"Huh?" I mumbled. I was tired.

"That grape," he rejoined, "has more genes than you do. Well, really the grape plant."

"What are you talking about?" I stammered.

"A grape plant has about eight thousand more nonredundant genes than a human being." Zach replied confidently.

I had to google it. Sure enough, a grape plant has 30,434 genes, approximately 8,000 more than a human.[1] How could this possibly be? Humans are the most sophisticated life-forms on Earth. How could we have less genes than a small fruit?

My entire world view of my health was changing! I had learned that the nonhuman single-celled microbes in my gut had massive influence on my health. Now, I was discovering that my hard-coded genetics were far from the ultimate arbiter of my well-being.

Through my interviews with Dr. Bruce Lipton and Dr. Kara Fitzgerald, I began to realize that biology, and, by extension, health, didn't hinge so much on the number of genes. Rather, biological processes were mitigated by the various expressions of those genes. Further, genes expressed themselves differently based on the environment—the exposome! This new understanding of the role of genes upended not only my understanding of genetics but also the broader 20th-century paradigm of genetic determinism.

Genetic Determinism

Let's rewind 70 years or so. It was 1953. James Watson and Francis Crick barged into the Eagle Pub in Cambridge, England, and brashly proclaimed that they had discovered "the secret of life." There was justifiable reason to enjoy a pint or three for Watson and Crick (and the largely unheralded female British chemist Rosalind Franklin) had uncovered the structure of DNA, the chemical that encodes instructions for the building and replication of life.

Watson and Crick proposed that the DNA molecule was made up of two chains of nucleotides paired in such a way as to form a double helix. This spiral-staircase-like structure explained how the DNA molecule could replicate itself during cell division, enabling organisms to reproduce themselves with amazing accuracy except for the occasional mutation.

This monumental discovery propelled biology for five decades on a quest to unpack the basic building blocks of life. It informed a biological model that envisioned life as fixed, predetermined by the combination of nitrogen-containing base pairs, the sequence of which informs your specific genetic makeup. Biology became consumed by the idea that we could map the human genome and isolate every gene responsible for the production of every protein, every behavioral trait, and even every disease. This fixation culminated in the Human Genome Project.

Launched in October 1990, the Human Genome Project was the largest collaborative international scientific research project in history. Its goal was to identify, map, and sequence the entirety of the human genome.

Given our vast intellectual prowess (read: hubris) and the hundreds of thousands of proteins coursing through our veins, scientists justifiably presumed that this vast effort would likely map a robust six-figure genome.

However, when the tally was complete in 2004, the number of protein-coding genes in human beings totaled approximately 22,300, the same range as in other mammals.[2] We only modestly outscored a fruit fly, who boasts 14,000 genes and lives barely a month. Indeed, *Homo sapiens* (which translates as "wise human") have the same quantity of protein-coding genes as a guppy.

The Human Genome Project was a triumph in international scientific cooperation, and its results were integral to our understanding of human life. The mapping and sequence of human genomics open up the possibilities to identify the genetic variants that increase the risk for common diseases. Undoubtedly, there are variations known as single nucleotide polymorphisms (SNPs) that predispose a person to disease. For example, sickle cell disease is a genetic disorder caused by a mutation in both copies of a person's HBB gene. Mutations in the BRCA1 gene are associated with an increased risk of breast cancer. Two copies of the APOE4 allele render a person 8 to 10 times more likely to develop late-onset Alzheimer's disease.[3]

All this said, the scant number of human genes raised as many questions as it answered.

How do we make hundreds of thousands of proteins from only 22,000 genetic recipes? Why do some people with the BRCA1 mutation get cancer and others don't? How and why do some genes "decide" to express themselves and others do not?

Just like Newtonian physics sought to find the universe's smallest component parts as a means to explain the nature of reality, many biologists believed that DNA held a similar promise. But, just as Einstein found that matter consisted of patterns of energy in constant flux and relationship, and just as Buddha posited his theory of impermanence and dependent origination in which everything changes in relation to everything else, modern biology points to the same satori.

We are not fixed beings with predetermined, hard-coded fates. We are fluctuating forms, changing in relation to our environment and behavior. The ebb of genetic determinism and the rising tide of epigenetics, neuroplasticity, and the microbiome have ushered in a paradigm shift. We have entered a new "age of agency." It is incredibly empowering—and, as I will explain, a little scary.

Epigenetics

Let me explain epigenetics by analogy with my first-ever public piano performance last spring.

I peeked through the curtain at the milling crowd. My palms immediately got clammy, and my heart started racing. But I did a little box breathing backstage and arrived on stage without any nerves.

I sat at my old, rickety 1970s Wurlitzer piano and beheld the keys. There they were, exactly as I had left them. I ran my fingers up a chromatic scale, starting on A and ending on G#. The notes never change, but I do. At times, I am relaxed, open, and dexterous; at other times, I am stiff, closed, and clunky.

The piano player—me, in this case—is the epigenome. He or she sits above the keys and influences their expression. My DNA is like the 88 keys on a piano. It's the hand I've been dealt, warts and all. But what keys will I "turn on"? And will they produce clusters of harmonious tones, or will they drive people from the club in their dissonance? You'll be happy to know that I delivered a most acceptable performance.

Here's the bigger headline: Our DNA predisposes us to certain conditions—on occasion, definitively. But the role that genes play as it pertains to chronic disease is diminishing. Epigenetics, the expression of our genes in relation to our environment, has now taken center stage. Our genes are expressed like a piece of music, and this expression can be adaptive or maladaptive. For example, tumor-suppressor genes can turn on in response to specific nutrients. A well-rested, destressed, properly fed pianist will leverage the keys at his disposal for beauty and coherence. The same is true of our bodies.

Epi means above. Genetics refer to my coding, or genome. Epigenetics, then, is what exists "above my genes," which is why sometimes I call it muffin tops, because my ever-diminishing muffin tops rest above my jeans. (TMI meets bad dad joke #xxx)

The term *epigenetics* gets used in two different, but related, ways. The primary definition of epigenetics, as stated, is the study of how gene expression modifies in relationship to behavior and the environment. The auxiliary definition of epigenetics refers to the transgenerational inheritance of acquired traits. In the latter sense, proponents of epigenetics theorize that certain characteristics that are acquired in response to experiences and environmental circumstances can be passed down to the next generation. I am only addressing the former definition here.

It turns out that lifestyle factors can impact epigenetic patterns. Diet, obesity, physical activity, tobacco smoking, alcohol consumption, environmental pollutants, psychological stress—all these inputs can change how your genes express themselves.

To best understand the nature of epigenetics, let's have a quick refresher on genetics.

You possess DNA that you inherit from your biological mother and father. There are four nitrogen-containing bases that pair up to form the fixed nucleotide sequences of your DNA. These are adenine (A), cytosine (C), guanine (G), and thymine (T). These bases form specific pairs (A with T, and G with C). It's the combination of these bases that creates the underlying code that determines your morphology—skin, hair, and eye color, among other traits.

Your DNA is wrapped in a protein called histone and organized along 23 pairs of chromosomes that exist in the nucleus of every human cell in your body (with the exception of red blood cells). These chromosomes house your genes.

Your genes provide the recipes for producing proteins, the codes for how to sequence amino acid building blocks. We often associate protein with muscle. And, it's true, our genes have the transcriptions for the growth of muscular structure known as hypertrophy. But proteins wear many cloaks of identity. They can be antibodies, contractile proteins, enzymes, hormonal proteins, structural proteins, storage proteins, and transport proteins.

Here's a way to think about it. The DNA is the master cookbook locked inside the inner sanctum of the nucleus. It contains the secret formulas. These recipes provide the proper sequencing of amino acids, the ingredients. These recipes are messengered out of the nucleus and into the kitchen of the cytoplasm. The ribosomes are the line cooks. They receive the recipes and then make the dish. Ribosomes link amino acids together in the order specified by the codes of messenger RNA molecules to form chains of amino acids that we know as peptides and proteins.

But what's on the menu tonight? Well, that's the job of the head chef, of course. He determines what recipes will make the specials menu. In this manner, the chef is the epigenome. He turns genes on and off. The chef is, in turn, influenced by many environmental factors. These ever-changing dynamics determine whether or not the restaurant (your body) is a smashing success or shutters prematurely.

How Does This All Work?

DNA methylation is one of the most common mechanisms in epigenetics. It involves the addition of a methyl group (one carbon atom bonded to three hydrogen atoms) to the DNA molecule, usually at a cytosine nucleotide.

This molecule, which curiously resembles a lollipop, connects to a gene promoter, a region of the DNA sequence that initiates transcription of a particular gene. This tryst generally leads to repression or the "silencing" of that gene. This is because the methyl groups prevent the transcription factors and other proteins required for transcription from accessing the DNA and initiating the process.

Hypermethylation, therefore, refers to the excessive methylation of certain genes. This can lead, for example, to the silencing of tumor-suppressor genes, which can potentially lead to the development and progression of cancer.

For instance, the hypermethylation of promoter regions in BRCA1, a gene associated with breast and ovarian cancer risk, can silence the gene, disabling its tumor-suppressing properties and increasing the risk of cancer.[4]

But, again, we are not fixed. Epigenetic changes are reversible. It is possible to turn genes back on that have been silenced by hypermethylation.

Chronological Age vs. Biological Age

I was born in 1970, so, as I sit here typing, my chronological age is 53. Chronological age is reflective of the number of orbits you've traveled around the sun, the number of candles on your gluten- and dairy-free birthday cake. Chronological age is a fixed value.

Biological age, on the other hand, is a measure of how well a person's physiological systems are functioning compared to others of the same chronological age. Biological age can be estimated in several ways, including through measures of cardiovascular fitness, telomere length, and more recently through the Horvath clock, which measures DNA methylation patterns.

The original Horvath clock, named after its creator Dr. Steve Horvath and published in 2013, uses the methylation status of 353 specific sites on the DNA molecule to estimate biological age. This estimate is often referred to as "epigenetic age" or "methylation age."

Since the development of the original Horvath clock, other DNA methylation-based age estimators have been developed. Some of these newer clocks are designed to predict not just age, but also healthspan, lifespan, or risk of specific age-related diseases.

I first tested my bio-age in 2018. My solar orbits totaled 48 but, sadly, my bio-age came back at 55. This means my body was functioning as well as the average 55-year-old. Further, "average" in this day and age is certainly not optimal. Stress, insomnia, a mediocre diet, and too much drinking had downregulated the expression of my genes.

Five years later, after applying the Good Stress protocols I will outline, my bio-age is now 45. My chronological age increased 5 years while my biological age decreased 10 years. By changing my behavior and my environment, my gene expression improved.

Why Do Genes Get Methylated?

Methylation patterns change naturally as we age. Some areas of the genome tend to become hypermethylated as we hurtle around the sun, while others may become hypomethylated. These fluctuations can influence the aging process and contribute to the development of age-related diseases.

More and more, however, we are discovering that environmental factors play a significant role in DNA methylation patterns, often leading to changes in gene expression. For example, certain nutrients directly supply the methyl groups needed for DNA methylation. These include folate, choline, and other B vitamins. Diets that are deficient in these nutrients could potentially affect DNA methylation patterns. I will share some of Dr. Kara Fitzgerald's work on epi-nutrition in Part II.

Toxins, such as heavy metals including lead, arsenic, and mercury, can lead to changes in gene expression. Lifestyle factors like smoking, alcohol consumption, and physical activity levels have all been linked with changes in DNA methylation patterns. For example, smoking has been associated with hypermethylation of certain genes, which could potentially contribute to the development of diseases like cancer. Both physical and psychological stress can lead to changes in DNA methylation. This is part of the reason why severe or prolonged stress is often associated with poor health outcomes.

Again, while our DNA may be static, gene expression is patently not fixed. This idea of being unfixed is both empowering and a little scary. Empowering because you have agency. You are a participant in your own well-being. Scary because your life is not just your own. Your health is inextricably tied to its environment whose inputs alter your gene expression.

We are all in flux—caught up in a mutually interdependent net of humanity—in constant relationship with everything and everyone around us.

I was beginning to build a foundational understanding for health.

Key Learnings:

1. The body is a process.
2. Ease and disease are not permanent states. They exist across a spectrum.
3. The behavior of your body is inseparable from the behavior and function of its environment.
4. Thus, healing and ailing are largely determined by one's exposome.
5. We have significant agency over our exposome—our environment and behavior.

CHAPTER 7

THE TAO OF HEALTH PRINCIPLE #4

Balance (the Teeter-Totter)

The equilibrium of nature is not a status quo but a ceaseless struggle among species for a niche advantage, which results in a fine-tuning and a convergence towards a middle ground in every ecological system.

— E.O. Wilson

If my organism is a process inseparable from my environment, then what is the key to optimal health?

Let me answer this question through the story of my first love, Sara.

I was two and a half. She was three. We met at a playground in the picturesque town of Santiago de Compostela, Spain, where I lived with my parents in 1973. I was smitten with her. Like a deal requires a buyer and a seller, so does love depend on a recipient and a provider. Sara was definitely the beloved, and I was the lover.

Our first date, and every other date, transpired on a rusting teeter-totter. She rested daintily on one side of the long board and I plunked down on the other, a fulcrum between us. Despite her being my elder, I had more heft. My weightiness, unchivalrously, shot her up in the air, as I plopped to ground level.

From my position as a lowly sentry, I gazed up at my lofty princess longingly. It was abundantly clear by the panicked look in her eyes, however, that she did not enjoy her exalted status. Gallantly, I focused on making myself lighter, instinctually shifting my weight inward toward the handles and then thrusting up mightily from my heels.

With this action, I jetted up and she went down, but too precipitously. She bounced rather violently on the hard-packed clay beneath her. And then, quite abruptly, gravity flexed its biceps and, to her dismay, up again she went.

This time, I took a gentle approach and pushed up delicately from my crouch. The plank settled on its pivot, parallel to the ground. She looked at me, and a big smile came across her face. We rested there for too little time, in a tenuous but perfect balance.

This must be love, I thought, the moment on the seesaw when no one's feet are touching the ground.

The Principle of Balance

Balance is a protean concept. It may refer to a condition in which different elements are in the correct proportions such as the balance of ingredients in a stew. It may also connote an even distribution of weight enabling something—like a seesaw—to remain steady.

Balance may refer to the relative volume of various sources of sound. There's a knob for balance on a stereo system—if you remember what that is. Depicted by the zodiac sign Libra, a balance is also an apparatus for weighing matters ranging from turmeric to justice. Balance can be a counteracting force or even a majority opinion.

Balance can also be a verb. You can balance a hot cup of coffee on your knee, though I don't recommend it. You can balance the worth of one thing with another, like the time value of money. And you can attempt, generally in vain, to balance your checkbook or work and family life.

Balance, as applied to myriad areas of life, both fosters and reflects healthy systems. In economics, balance is represented by a thriving middle class. In nature, through biodiversity. In our body politic, by cooperation and compromise. When systems cluster toward the center, they are generally healthy.

Of course, balance is also fundamental to human well-being—spiritually, psychologically, and physiologically.

The concept of balance echoes across the mystical traditions of the East. In Buddhism, balance is encapsulated by the middle way, originally the path to enlightenment between hedonism and asceticism.

Taoism understands balance as the foundational intelligence of nature itself. Balance in nature occurs between countervailing forces. The natural world arises as a coincidence of opposites. Up and down (as depicted). Hot and cold. Right and left. Hard and soft. Strong and supple. Being and nonbeing. And, yes, lover and beloved.

According to Taoism, the fundamental intelligence of nature brings opposites into balance. However, the balance induced by nature is like that of a seesaw. It is unstable. If you've ever tried to balance on a slackline, then you know its precarity as a product of direct experience.

Balance in nature is a dynamic and ever-changing process that requires constant adaptation and adjustment. Of course, your organism *is* nature, and it innately seeks out balance—a sensitive type of asymmetrical order that is perpetually influenced, for better and worse, by its environment.

The universe, along with your organism, is in a constant state of spontaneous emergence. It is an endless succession of simultaneous chemical reactions. Everything is in flux, constructing and deconstructing. Therefore, trying to hold on to a fixed position or state is futile, because it is impossible to evade the impermanence of life. Perfect balance can only be momentarily glimpsed. You see it and it's gone.

Thus, balance is not about finding a perfect state but about refining your skill to navigate the ups and downs of life with thoughtfulness and equanimity. It is about being in tune with the rhythms of nature, aligning yourself with its intelligence, and being able to flow with the current of life, rather than resisting or trying to swim upstream.

Your body's literal balance, spatial orientation, and coordination is maintained curiously in your ear. The vestibular system is a complex network of structures, canals and fluids that detect gravity, acceleration and tilt and deliver this information to the brain. It works closely with other sensory apparati, such as the visual system and proprioception, your body's sense of its own position in space, to help you walk to the coffee maker without falling over. Given my love of espresso, I am eternally grateful for this feat of engineering.

Psychologically, balance points to the stability of one's mind or feelings. We endeavor to cultivate a serene mind, one not pulled too dramatically to the thinner edges. We attempt to avoid over-assigning advantage or disadvantage to any situation. We try to see events for what they are and not be emotionally swayed by our judgments of them. We often call this equipoise "being centered."

Physiologically, we strive for a balanced immune system, for hormonal balance, and for balanced blood sugar. In fact, virtually every system of human physiology is an exercise in balancing opposing activities and nurturing a sensitive equilibrium.

Balance in your organism is called homeostasis, the moment on the seesaw when no one's feet are touching the ground.

Bouncing Back

Your body is programmed to seek out balance in the most astounding ways and to recalibrate when imbalances occur. We often think about this as "bouncing back."

You experience this bouncing back all the time. You sprint up a hill or have an uncommonly enthusiastic roll in the hay (perhaps more rarely). In response, your heart and breath rate spike. And then when you "consummate" the activity, within minutes, your respiratory rate naturally decelerates to between 12–16 breaths per minute,[1] and your heart rate finds the warm porridge of 60–80.[2]

To bounce back refers to the body's ability to recover from imbalances. This concept is often used in the context of resilience in the face of the inevitable challenges and setbacks of life. Indeed, our ability to return to a previous state of equilibrium may be the greatest measure of our well-being.

This recalibration is relentlessly occurring under the crust of consciousness. Our bodies thermoregulate in response to decreases or increases in core body temperature. We generate heat or perspire to bring ourselves back into the Goldilocks zone, around 98.6. Our bodies maintain a delicate acid-alkaline pH balance, around 7.4. The liver titrates with great precision to maintain balanced blood glucose levels of around 90 mg/dL.[3] Fluid-electrolyte balance, blood pressure regulation, hormone counter-regulation . . . the dance of homeostasis is happening everywhere.

Bouncing back is not only the province of the physiological. Life continually tests our ability to recover from distressing and traumatic experiences. We confront failure, criticism, and disappointment. Through processing negative emotions and finding meaning and growth in challenges, we regain our balance. We find our center. We bounce back.

Ironically, as I will describe, the deliberate application of stress in the right doses enhances the ability of the body-mind to recalibrate. In this manner, stress of a particular variety is an opportunity. The Good Stress protocols that I will describe foster balance. They help you "bounce back."

If ease in the body is a product of balance, then dis-ease arises when the body and mind cease to be able to bounce back to homeostasis.

A Coincidence of Opposites

Once we perceive beauty in the world,
we also discern ugliness.
After we gain knowledge of goodness,
we also recognize evil.
Existence and the void give birth to each other.
Difficult and easy determine each other.
Long and short measure each other.
High and low position each other.
Tone and silence
make melodies together.
Before and after
march in the same parade.

— Lao Tzu, *Tao Te Ching*, Verse 2

Have you ever seen a person with a front and no back? Have you ever been on an elevator that only goes up? Can there be an ending without a beginning? Would you even be able to determine what is hot without experiencing cold?

If you answered yes to any of these questions, well, then you are quite strange. But how would I even know "strange" without knowing "normal"?

All phenomena in the universe inherently exist as a *coincidentia oppositorum*—a coincidence of opposites—that arise mutually.

Up. Down. Right. Left. Front. Back. Hot. Cold. Day. Night. Sun. Moon. Summer. Winter. Wakefulness. Sleep. Abundance. Scarcity. Male. Female. Fire. Water. Growth. Repair.

This coincidence of opposites is represented by the ancient Chinese symbol the yin-yang, the origin of which relates to the sunny and shady sides of a mountain. You cannot have a sunny face without a shady face. And this coexistence creates a great irony. The duality of opposites, like sunniness and shadiness, points to an ultimate non-duality. This paradox is known as the unity of opposites. The unity of opposites defines a situation in which the existence of a thing or situation depends on the simultaneity of at least two conditions that are opposite to each other, yet reliant on each other.

For example, "sunny" cannot exist unless there is a "shady." They are opposites, but they co-substantiate one another. Their unity is that either one exists because the opposite is necessary for the existence of the other. One condition instantiates the other.

Hot could not be hot without cold, as a result of there being no contrast by which to define it as "hot" relative to any other condition. Hot could not have its identity if not for its opposite. The existence of hot and cold respectively are bound to each other. Hot is a prerequisite for cold and vice versa.

A deal implies a seller and a buyer. And, in this sense, your body is a "deal"—brimming with mutually arising countervailing forces—at once explicitly distinct while implicitly unified.

Of course, opposites exist along a spectrum and in a constant state of flux. The sunny side of the mountain is not always sunny. At times, depending on the season, time of day, and position of the sun, the sunny side has a bit of shade. And, on the flip side, the shady side may have a dollop of sun on it.

This, too, is represented in the yin-yang, as the white of the yang has an eye of yin in it. And the black of yin has an eye of white in it.

The mutually dependent duality of the yin-yang sits atop of an empty circle known as tai chi, the ultimate reality, the emptiness from which the phenomenal world instantiates.

The mutual arising of opposites is everywhere to be found and is central to all forms of energy. Electricity is dependent on the attraction and repulsion of negatively and positively charged particles. Electromagnetic radiation exists as waves characterized by crests and troughs, amplitudes and frequencies. Sound energy also has a wave structure with amplitudes defining its volume and frequencies revealing its pitch. And, of course, hydraulics often have literal waves.

YIN-YANG

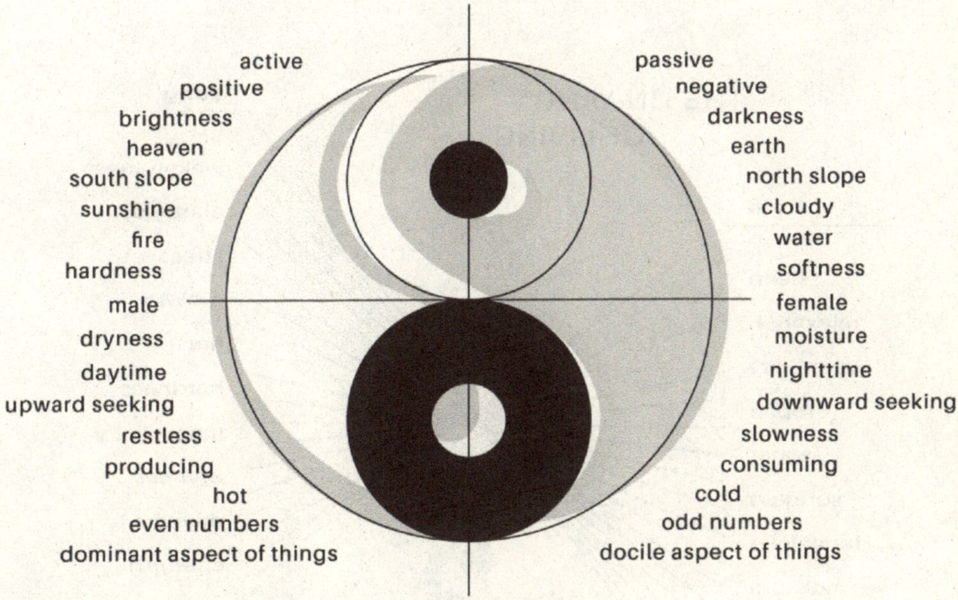

THE UNITY OF OPPOSITES

Nature, when unimpeded, brings opposites into a sensitive order. This is the foundational cosmic intelligence, the Tao, the force that pulls polarities into tenuous balance.

This very same concept can be applied to your body. The yin-yang of your physiology is omnipresent. Nearly every function, hormone, neurotransmitter, and cellular pathway has its counterpart. Your entire organism exists as a series of crests and troughs, yangs and yins.

Many of our physiological contrapositions are hidden in plain sight. Growth, wakefulness, alertness, extraversion, and pleasure reflect our yang. Repair, sleep, dreaminess, introversion, and serenity suggest our yin. These states sit atop of mechanisms—on/off switches that are on a dimmer. One state rarely exists without a glimmer of its opposing state. And, when it does, there is generally a significant imbalance. Even strength must have some suppleness as depicted by the branches of a willow that will bend flexibly under the load of a heavy snow. This limberness allows the snow to slough off, where the stiff boughs of an oak may snap.

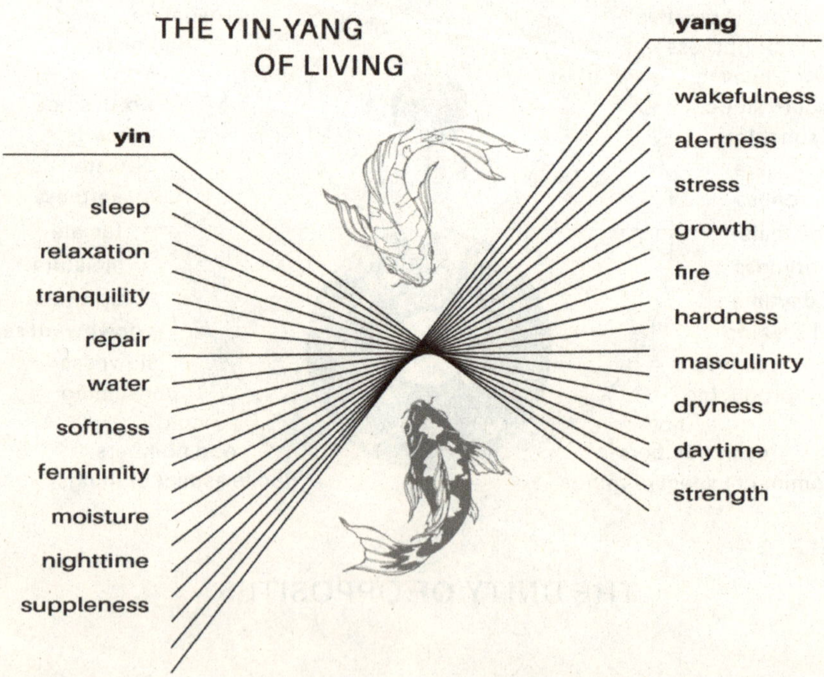

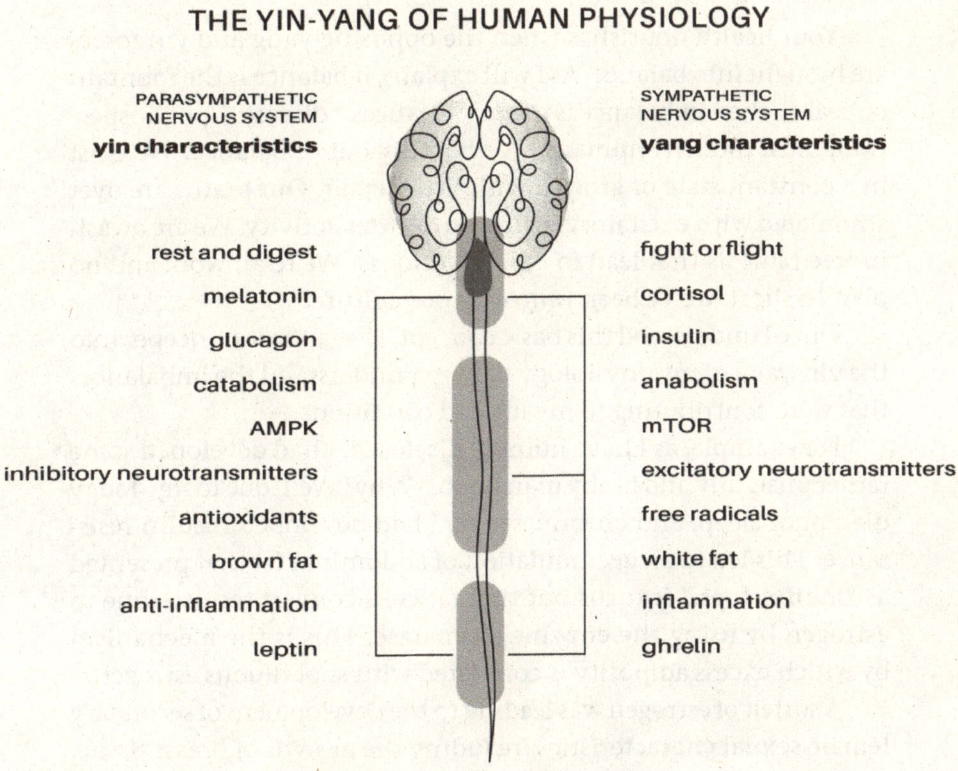

These broader oppositional characteristics of life are underwritten by specific counterposing molecules and pathways in the body.

I will explore many of these in depth in Part II. At the end of every chapter, I have included a section dubbed "The Body in Balance," which probes many of the counterregulatory molecules and systems in the human body. For example, there are growth pathways like mTOR and repair pathways like AMPK. There are excitatory neurotransmitters like glutamate and inhibitory neurotransmitters like GABA. There are molecules known as free radicals who are counterposed by antioxidants.

The wholesale categorization of molecules as either yin or yang is an oversimplification, but the taxonomy is not without merit. The classification helps us to understand the essentialism of balance.

We've Been Yanged!

Your health flourishes when the opposing yang and yin forces are brought into balance. As I will explain, if balance is the fountain of health, then imbalance is the provenance of disease. Upon inspection, most modern humans are wickedly out of balance. We exist in a constant state of growth with little repair. Our brains are over stimulated with excitatory neurotransmitter activity. We are awash in free radicals that lead to oxidative stress. We're all work and no play. In short, we've been *yanged* by our culture!

Once I understood this basic concept, I began to look deeper into the yin-yang of my physiology to better understand the imbalances that were contributing to my myriad conditions.

For example, as I have humbly disclosed, I had developed some rather unsightly and fleshy man boobs. Why? Well, due to my dodgy diet, poor sleep, and chronic stress, I had developed insulin resistance. This led to an accumulation of abdominal fat that presented as "muffin tops." It turns out that fat cells convert testosterone to estrogen by using the enzyme aromatase. This is the mechanism by which excess adiposity is correlated with superfluous estrogen.

A surfeit of estrogen was leading to the development of secondary female sexual characteristics including the growth of breast tissue. Hence, the boobs of man. Higher estrogen levels in men may also result in conditions that injure more than one's vanity, like prostate cancer.

You Put Your Yang in My Yin

In the iconic yin-yang symbol, there is a bit of one in the other. Strength actually requires a degree of suppleness, just as flexibility necessitates some firmness.

If the yin-yang of your body was adapted into a popular movie, the leading roles would almost certainly be filled by the hormones estrogen and testosterone. While it would be most obvious to cast estrogen as the female lead and testosterone as the male protagonist, both sexes have estrogen and testosterone in their bodies, just in different ratios. And the volume of each respective hormone changes due to a variety of circumstances.

As different as they are, these hormones share some common traits. Both estrogen and testosterone are steroid hormones, derived from cholesterol, a type of lipid found in all cells of the body. While you can consume dietary cholesterol, your body also synthesizes it endogenously at the cellular level.

So, while testosterone is an androgen and often dubbed the "male hormone," women also require a dollop of the yang hormone. And while estrogen is often labeled the "female hormone," men also require the right amount of it.

Let me further illustrate this concept briefly by looking at another set of oppositional hormones, ghrelin and leptin. Before doing so, let me provide the briefest primer on hormones.

Hormones are the body's homing pigeons, flying through the bloodstream, carrying messages to your organs, skin, and muscles. These chemical signals tell your body what to do and when to do it. Hormones and the glands that produce and release them make up your endocrine system and influence many different bodily processes including metabolism, blood sugar regulation, sexual function, sleep-wake cycle, growth, and development and mood. Scientists have identified approximately 50 hormones in the human body, but there are likely many more that we haven't yet put our thumb on.

Ghrelin vs. Leptin: More and Enough

Imagine two countervailing forces at play within your body, one that tells you when you are full and satisfied and another that tells you when you are hungry and in need of nourishment. Leptin and ghrelin are two peptide hormones that are involved in regulating the sensations of satiety and hunger in the body. In the best-case scenario, they seesaw back and forth. Ghrelin increases in the body as you sleep. And, after you've eaten, leptin signals your brain that you are sated.

The names leptin and ghrelin sound like characters out of Grimm's fairy tales. Leptin plays the part of the wise old sage, protecting you from overindulgence. It reminds you that you have eaten enough and have sufficient energy storage. Ghrelin, on the other hand, is the eager apprentice, urging you to seek out more fuel for your tank.

Leptin is produced by fat cells and is involved in regulating energy balance. It acts on the hypothalamus, a part of the brain that controls hunger and metabolism, to reduce appetite and increase energy expenditure. Leptin levels are typically higher in individuals who have more body fat.

While leptin is famously the "satiety" hormone, it might be better described as the signal that says "enough." Not just in the sense of "I've had enough dinner," but also in a manner that tells the brain that there is sufficient stockpiled energy within fat cells to take on colossal physical challenges, including childbearing.

Increased adiposity due to poor diet and sedentariness can lead to the overproduction of leptin. Just like guzzling a case of Budweiser every day will increase your tolerance for alcohol, the brain's tolerance threshold for leptin increases when it is delivered by the keg. Eventually, one can become leptin resistant, undermining the hormone's purpose. So, you become a hungry ghost who is never sated.

Adiposity and the overproduction of leptin might explain another disturbing phenomenon related to menarche, the onset of puberty. According to German researchers, the average age of a girl's first period in 1860 was 16.6 years.[4] The average age today is around 10.[5]

It is likely that "overnutrition" leading to the accumulation of more adipocytes in girls is partly responsible for this trend. Leptin is, in essence, giving the brain the message that there is enough stored energy in the body to meet the demands of pregnancy. In response, the brain triggers the processes that begin menstruation. Early menarche triggers the production of estrogen, which leads to the development of secondary sexual characteristics like widening hips and breast development. Increasingly, ten-year-old girls (and younger) are maturing arguably before they are psychologically ready. This sexualization of girls, particularly in the age of social media, can result in anxiety and eating disorders.

Ghrelin, on the other hand, is a hormone that is produced in the stomach and stimulates appetite. It acts on the same hypothalamic receptors as leptin, but has the opposite effect, increasing appetite and decreasing energy expenditure. Ghrelin levels logically increase before meals and decrease post prandially.

Ultimately, we must learn to foster balance in all aspects of our lives. By attuning with our bodies and adopting the appropriate mix of Good Stress protocols outlined in this book, we can foster that healthy, if tenuous, equilibrium that I had with Sara on the seesaw.

Key Learnings:

1. Health, in all of its expressions, arises from balance.
2. Balance is a sensitive, tenuous state of equilibrium.
3. Balance is the cultivation of equilibrium between opposing forces (yins and yangs).
4. Balance in the body is called homeostasis.
5. Your organism is full of counterposing molecules, processes, and systems.
6. Disease is a result of imbalance, failures to maintain homeostasis.

CHAPTER 8

CULTURE IS FAST. EVOLUTION IS SLOW.

Disease & Imbalance

Many of the problems we face in the modern industrialized world are not due to any fundamental defect in our nature but rather to a mismatch between the social world in which we now live and the social world for which our neural and physiological mechanisms were originally adapted.

— DANIEL NETTLE

Why are we so sick? Why are the rates of the FUCKs cresting like a mammoth wave? If imbalances in the body are the source of disease, what is the cause of these imbalances?

To excavate these questions and to make it a bit more enjoyable, let me introduce you to my distant East African ancestor, Ffej Onsark (my name spelled backward for those curious). Ffej lived as a hunter-gatherer, like his father and his father's father and his father's father's father, on the plains of what we now call Kenya some 12,000 years ago.

Ffej, like hundreds of generations before him and after him, endured significant environmental discomforts. He was an opportunistic omnivore, eating 800 different plants, seeds, tubers, and occasional wild game but was also forced to withstand periods of food scarcity. He bore bouts of extreme heat and cold, relying only on his internal thermostat to maintain temperature homeostasis. He walked and lifted heavy things. He lived communally and in nature, woke with the sun, squatted, and wore minimal shoes.

You could say Ffej lived with the H.I.P.P.I.E.S. (Health Imparting Paleolithic Period Inconvenient Environmental Stressors). Ffej's way of life was the norm for approximately 200,000 years and across this unfathomable swath of time, *Homo sapiens* evolved, developing adaptive mechanisms in relation to environmental adversity. Nature played its part, selecting for the traits most apt to foster physiological homeostasis and resilience.

Ffej and I share virtually the same exact biology. In fact, give him a shave and some jeans and walk him down Main Street, and no one even bats an eye. But while our genome may be virtually identical, the cultures in which we live could not be more different. And, of course, we cannot separate who we are from our environment. You and I live in an ecosystem characterized by the Big MACs. No, not just the ones you scarf down at the Evil M. I am speaking of the Big "modern American conveniences."

On a whim and from the palm of my hand, I can order up any type of ultra-processed foodstuff 365 days a year. I can get a summer squash delivered to my front door before you finish reading the next chapter—in the winter! Like most denizens of modernity, I sit sedentary at a desk for eight hours per day (writing this damn book) in a climate-controlled office. I inhabit a culture where it is the norm for humans to spend a mere 6 percent of our time outdoors and to live largely alone, often in gated communities, single-family homes or vertical boxes.[1] We enjoy 24-7 on-demand entertainment, wrap our feet in padded plastic and lounge about in cushy armchairs. We opt for wrinkle-free, stain-free, water-resistant, and nonstick wherever possible.

Over the past century and a half, our lifestyle has been engineered primarily for ease and convenience. In an evolutionary blink of an eye, culture has hijacked our adaptive mechanisms and rendered them maladaptive. The Big MACs—the overabundance of nutrient-deficient highly caloric food, our incessant eating cycle, blue light exposure, temperature neutrality, sedentariness, technology, individualism, and other creature comforts—have upended our hard-wrought evolutionary advantages.

Culture is fast. Evolution is slow.

Modernity has created a panoply of evolutionary mismatches that are making us sick. While it's true that Ffej's life expectancy was less than half of mine, the shorter average lifespan of hunter-gatherers was primarily due to infant mortality, the inability to treat infection, and the spread of communicable diseases. Indeed, modern medicine has made great progress in these respects.

However, no one in Ffej's tribe had heart disease or diabetes or dementia. Cancer was extremely rare. Fatty liver disease, kidney disease, autoimmune diseases, and mental disorders like ADHD, autism, PTSD, and others were virtually nonexistent.

If Ffej and we are "wearing the same genes," so to speak, why are we so sick with the chronic diseases? The answer is simple and obvious. It's our lifestyle. Our culture of chronic ease is creating an epidemic of chronic dis-ease.

Here is a smattering of our comfort-induced evolutionary mismatches and their knock-on impacts:

1. Modernity's constant feeding cycles hijack the body's programming to store energy resulting in obesity, diabetes, and heart disease.
2. Exposure to hormone-disrupting blue light in the evening results in insomnia.
3. Sedentariness results in sarcopenia, osteoporosis, and obesity.
4. Temperature neutrality results in low metabolic rate and decreased resilience.
5. Information overwhelm results in distraction, comparison, and an inability to concentrate.
6. Digital communication results in polarization and lack of cooperation.
7. Rampant individualism results in an epidemic of loneliness.

8. Industrial agriculture that grows nutrient-depleted food results in poor health.
9. Indoor living, comfortable shoes, easy chairs, and a divorce from nature results in muscle atrophy, poor immunity, lack of balance, and higher stress levels.

Of course, humans have always sought some degree of convenience. The mastery of fire opened nature's pantry, providing a surfeit of calories that led to the doubling of brain size. Humans also developed tools, weapons, and forms of shelter that provided protection from predation. We used animal hides to protect our feet from puncture and frostbite. Such advancements were typically slow and adaptive. In the last 150 years, however, cultural innovation—generally driven by economics—has jumped the perch of evolution.

There are two ways to solve for these evolutionary mismatches that have seen "survival of the fittest" morph into survival of the sickest. We can mask the symptoms of disease with expensive drugs and attempt technological moonshots to change our genetics in order to adapt to our culture. Or we can choose to "inconvenience" ourselves and realign our lifestyles with our biology by embracing the protocols of Good Stress.

In Part II, I make the case for the latter, for living a little more like Ffej.

Key Learnings:

1. Disease arises from imbalances, the inability to maintain homeostasis.
2. Imbalances are caused by the exposome—our environment and our behaviors.
3. Our culture—the way we have shaped our environment—produces imbalances.
4. To re-instill balance, we need to realign our culture—the way we live—with our biology.

Part II

THE PROTOCOLS OF GOOD STRESS

What to Do?

CHAPTER 9

WHAT IS GOOD STRESS?

Out of life's school of war:
What doesn't kill me makes me stronger.
— Friedrich Nietzsche

At first blush, this 1888 aphorism from German philosopher Friedrich Nietzsche appears as absurd as the Kelly Clarkson pop hit that quoted it. When I was 13, I had a malignant tumor on my left knee and spent three weeks at Memorial Sloan Kettering Cancer Center. Apparently, it didn't kill me. But how, exactly, did it make me stronger?

It wasn't until I began probing the cerebra of Mark Hyman, Wim Hof, Sara Gottfried, Will Cole, Andrew Huberman, and others that I got greater insight into Nietzsche's adage. These interviews revealed that a key to fostering homeostasis and well-being was the deliberate application of good old paleolithic stress.

You might justifiably ask yourself, "Why would I want to live more like Ffej? Hunter-gatherer life seems awfully onerous. I've got enough 'stress' in my life."

Indeed, life was demanding for Ffej Onsark on the Serengeti. Ffej endured periods of food scarcity and exposure to wide-ranging temperature fluctuations. Intense physical labor was a customary part of daily life. He had little if any shelter and minimal shoes at best. As if being responsible for his own welfare wasn't difficult enough, Ffej also shouldered the well-being of the greater tribe.

However, these paleolithic stressors differ greatly from the manner in which we generally experience stress in the twenty-first century.

For years at Wanderlust, I stressed over budgets. Indeed, most of the time, we *were* over budget. I stressed over the incoming asteroid field of e-mails and texts and Slacks and calls. I stressed about money—and whether I'd have enough to deliver the promise of America's dream to my children. I stressed about "being successful" generally through the eyes of everyone else.

My methods for assuaging this stress—late-night burritos and cabernet varietals—provided short-term reprieve but only compounded my anxiety day to day. My psychotherapy became Amazon Prime, an affordable option, but stress relief via retail indulgence was also only ephemeral. My methods of self-comfort generally were maladaptive. I was "de-stressing" myself into insomnia, corpulence, agitation, and, eventually, diabetes. My plight is not uncommon.

Modern stress is a chronic IV drip that contributes to the slow progressive onset of disease. Stress on the Serengeti, on the contrary, generally came in quick bursts and activated protective physiological mechanisms that promoted resilience. Ffej would occasionally flee from a predator, brave periods of food paucity, dip in a cold stream, and withstand stints of brutally high temperatures. Too much cold led to hypothermia and could be fatal. Too much extended heat could lead to heatstroke. But, as Paracelsus, the Swiss physician quipped, "the dose makes the poison." The right level of stress has become known as "eustress" and elicits hormesis, a positive psychological or physiological response to adversity.

This phenomenon has informed a variety of protocols sometimes known as adversity mimetics. These praxes *center* the body-mind. They foster a middle way, as they bring imbalances back into the sensitive balance that promotes well-being.

Let me clearly delineate between "good" acute stress and "bad" chronic stress.

Last week, I went for a hike in Fryman Canyon to clear my head prior to conducting a podcast interview. The narrow, serpentine hiking trail snakes along the side of a steep grade of chaparral. As I looped back toward home, I heard a rustling in the bramble. And then, quite suddenly, a coyote bounded out of the thicket and plunked into the middle of the trail some 10 yards in front of me. He fixed his eyes on me intently.

Startled, I stopped in my tracks. My heart began pounding. I felt a surge of adrenaline course through my veins. My lungs pumped. My eyes focused. Underneath the crust of consciousness, my adrenals were releasing cortisol that, in turn, messaged my liver to release glucose to power my muscles to flee (and, in this circumstance, not fight). But I didn't take flight. I just stood my ground. The coyote paused momentarily, and, realizing that I wouldn't be lunch, he slinked down the hill and out of sight. Within a minute or two, my heart and breath rate returned to normal. And, with a little pep in my step, I scampered home. This experience reflects a standard adaptive stress response. The stress came and went.

My rendezvous with Mr. Coyote represents an acute, short-term type of stress. Acute stress can either be thrilling (like riding a roller coaster) or distressing (like narrowly avoiding a car accident). It's the body's immediate involuntary response to a perceived threat, challenge, or scare—the classic fight-or-flight response. This type of stress is typically resolved quickly and doesn't have time to do the extensive damage associated with long-term stress. In many cases, acute stress, as we will see, is actually beneficial.

Chronic stress, on the other hand, is a state of ongoing physiological arousal. This condition occurs when the body experiences stressors with such consistency or intensity that the autonomic nervous system does not have a chance to activate the relaxation response. The coyote never leaves; rather, it stalks you. You never return to homeostasis.

Chronic "distress" can be due to ongoing pressures, such as work deadlines, sustained heavy workloads, family tumult, or poverty, but it can also be attributable to traumatic experiences. Chronic stress can lead to serious health problems, including the FUCKs: heart disease, cancer, diabetes, and dementia.

Good stress, or eustress, is a form of *deliberate* acute short-term stress. This is the type of stress I set out to explore as a means to address my litany of infirmities. I adopted dual roles as amateur biologist and willing, if sometimes reticent, subject of my experimentation. I tampered and tinkered with many protocols until I saw results. In my search to become healthy, I began to examine my behaviors through the lens of this question: How did I evolve? And how do I align my life with evolution's wisdom?

Across four years, I harvested the adversity practices that led me back to well-being and codified them as Good Stress.

You can think of them as the protocols of inconvenience to meet a world obsessed with convenience.

The following chapters chronicle this journey. I unpack the practices, the science behind them, their etiologies, their conferred benefits, and their recommended dosages. I focus primarily on the "ancient" stressors as, in most instances, these represent the natural conditions in which we evolved. Instilling Good Stress realigns the way I live with my evolutionary adaptations.

Old & True

Before (good) stressing you out, however, I *must* tell you about this *new* modality that can relieve anxiety, lower blood sugar, grow cortical thickness, and upregulate your immune system! I read about it in *The New York Times*. It's called . . . meditation. Everybody's doing it!

I jest, of course, but in interview after interview with everyone from sleep experts to neuroscientists, from immunologists to psychotherapists, from weight loss experts to athletic trainers, I kept hearing the same prescriptions to address a wide range of disorders.

Meditation, breathwork, yoga, movement, spending time in nature, deliberate cold and heat immersion, and fasting were among the most common recommended therapies.

You'll notice quickly that these modalities aren't actually novel at all. Yoga is 4,000 years old.[1] Conscious breathing practices (pranayama) dates back 5,000 years to the Upanishads.[2] Meditation is likely older. Fasting has been leveraged therapeutically since at least the 5th century B.C.E., when Greek physician Hippocrates recommended abstinence from food or drink for patients who exhibited certain symptoms of illness. Further, many of these protocols were inseparable from pre-Abrahamic spiritual traditions. Once upon a time, medicine and mysticism were merged, for better and, occasionally, for worse.

The paleo diet, which emerged in the 1970s and came into vogue in the early aughts as a weight loss method, is . . . well . . . paleolithic. In other words, it is 2.5 million years old. The ketogenic low-carbohydrate diet was a rather easy option on the Serengeti given the absence of 7-Elevens, minimarts, and other repositories for refined sugars and starches. Cold-water therapy dates back to 2500 B.C.E. to the ancient Egyptians, who leveraged its application to reduce inflammation and as an analgesic.[3] Heat therapy has taken on myriad historical secular and spiritual forms, including Native American sweat lodges, ancient Roman and Turkish baths, and Islamic hammams.

Wilding, grounding, walking barefoot, and forest bathing simply mimic the way humans existed in nature for tens of thousands of years. Tai chi, Qigong, acupuncture, cupping, and herbal remedies are relics of China and traditional Chinese medicine that go back 5,000 years.[4]

Sleep hygiene, which most prominently consists of getting blue light in the morning in order to set your circadian rhythm, was simply a product of sleeping outdoors or in small huts and waking with the sun.

"Local and organic food" is merely what foragers ate for hundreds of thousands of years. Regenerative farming techniques were quite "conventional" across the agricultural revolution.

The reason why all these ancient modalities function so well today is because they calibrate our style of life with the adaptive mechanisms that have been a product of hundreds of thousands of years of evolution.

At the risk of being redundant, the problem is that humanity has jumped the perch of evolution, particularly over the past 150 years. Chronic diseases are actually cultural infirmities. In the following chapters, I will describe the specific ways in which chronic ease has produced chronic disease and the Good Stress protocols that realign us with our own engineering and foster vibrancy and balance.

There are, of course, newfangled deliberate stressors like ozone therapy, hyperbaric chambers, and cryotherapy. These praxes are the darlings of biohackers and may be very beneficial, if, at times, pricey. Amortalists such as Bryan Johnson and Dave Asprey address these options with aplomb. But I concentrate on the old and true (and mostly free), including:

- Intermittent fasting
- Deliberate cold therapy
- Deliberate heat therapy
- Resistance training
- Light therapy
- Mind training & the breath
- Building psychological immunity
- Social fitness
- Eating stressed plants
- Rewilding

These are the praxes I slowly adopted and carefully stacked over the course of three years. This catalog of activities might actually come off as quite anodyne. I'm not ascending Mount Everest, swimming the English Channel, living in an ashram, or water fasting for weeks. In fact, over time, these "stressors" ceased to be particularly stressful at all. Yet they all have specific purposes and mechanisms attached to them.

These specific praxes are not the *only* way. They are just *my* way. But, like it or probably not, we share a common biology. As I mentioned earlier, all human beings are 99.9 percent identical in their genetic makeup. Despite our bio-individualities, some homogenous generalities apply.

These protocols have yielded uncommonly good results for me. I've tamed the wild tiger of my blood sugar, reversing my insulin resistance. I've largely curbed my insomnia, which has been my Achilles' heel for much of my adult life. My chronological age is 54 as of this moment but, according to numerous tests, my bio-age—which measures the health of my cells—is 45. My energy levels and stamina are stellar. My biomarkers all fall within the optimal ranges. And I've summoned enough focus—just barely—to put down my phone and pen this book.

By adopting the practices that I outline (of course, in consultation with your doctor), you too can jump into your own petri dish, be your own N-of-1 experiment, and experience the joy of self-transformation.

The sequence of these chapters doesn't necessarily reflect the importance of each protocol. They all contribute to holistic health. That said, I start with fasting, cold (and heat) therapy, and resistance training, as these were the primary tools I used to reverse my insulin resistance and improve my metabolic markers.

Some of these protocols have contraindications. For example, you may not want to fast if you are menstruating or pregnant. If you have some form of cardiovascular disease, you'll want to be cautious about deliberate heat or cold therapy. If we're to faithfully follow Nietzsche's axiom, in order to be stronger, we must not kill ourselves!

Still, all these protocols are scientifically proven to confer health benefits if applied in the right circumstances with the proper dosage. You'll just want to ease into the ones that best work for you. Let me "stress" this point. You don't begin a cold therapy practice by jumping into 34-degree water or start a fasting protocol with a week-long water fast. Instead, you walk slowly and consciously into these practices and take them day by day.

So, how did my adolescent stint in the hospital make me stronger? Well, that's likely the subject of another book but, in short, doing hard things makes doing other hard things easier. Through adversity, you build resilience—in both body and mind.

CHAPTER 10

HUMANS ARE DESIGNED TO BE FAT (JUST NOT ALL THE TIME)

Fasting

Fasting is the first principle of medicine;
fast and see the strength of the spirit reveal itself.
— Rumi

In January 2020, I organized a fundraiser for Marianne Williamson at Wanderlust Hollywood, a fantastic multistory wellness venue that I built in Los Angeles. At the time, Marianne was a Democratic candidate for the president of the United States. Before Commune's website was even live, Marianne agreed to shoot the first course for the platform in my living room in Laurel Canyon. As a result, I've always felt indebted to her. The "new" need friends. And she was a good one. In the spirit of reciprocity, I signed on to raise money for her fledgling campaign.

The evening featured Marianne in conversation with comedian-cum-spiritualist-cum-political commentator Russell Brand. I was looking after Russell's career at that juncture, a pursuit that I wouldn't categorize as *good* stress. Our work together focused on recovery from addiction as applied to drugs, alcohol, pornography, shopping, gambling, though patently not coffee. The night of the event arrived and, a dozen espresso shots later, I got Russell to the side of the stage.

As master of ceremonies, I subdued the butterflies fluttering in my substantial gut to deliver a rousing oratory introducing our guests of honor. The event was a smashing success. I glad-handed the glitterati and potential donors until the last Tesla silently slid out the parking lot.

The echoes of "Marianne! Marianne!" were now but attenuated whispers. A couple of shoe-printed handbills were strewn about the floor. And, like thousands of nights before, I stood in the alpenglow of the mayhem, head spinning and alone. And I did what I always did. I sought out food and drink to reward my efforts and calm my frazzled nerves.

Oddly, Los Angeles does not offer a glut of late-night eateries like other cities. With the options limited, I soon found myself at a Denny's at the junction of Gower and Sunset. I snuggled into a corner booth and ordered a beer with only a miniscule pang of guilt. My work in the recovery space certainly didn't apply to myself. I perused the sandwich board that was affixed above the counter. I was both scandalized, and momentarily pleased, to discover that there were now four meals per day—at least at Denny's—including breakfast (served all day, thank God!), lunch, dinner, and . . . late night!

Hmmm, I thought to myself. *We're hungry ghosts. We never stop eating.* And, then, I proceeded to order a turkey club.

I rolled out of Denny's stuffed and transiently relaxed. Food provided me with a type of fleeting relief. This phenomenon is a confection of a broader devil's bargain: short-term comfort in exchange for long-term discomfort.

I got home, lumbered into bed, and fell immediately asleep only to awaken at 2:45 A.M. and cash in my REM slumber for another bout of early morning tossing and turning. Fortunately, once again, there was espresso. This pattern of behavior eventually manifested in diabetes.

I would discover through my many interviews that our modern incessant eating cycle is at loggerheads with our biology. As I have described, you cannot separate the individual from its environment.

Over millennia, food scarcity has shaped the development of human physiology. I am simply the delegated adaptability of a process called evolution. My genes are a product of nature's inherent cycles of abundance and paucity.

However, it wasn't poring over Satchin Panda's clinical research on fasting that initially inspired me to break my continuous eating cycle. It was another set of dusty scrolls that propelled me to time restrict my eating.

While most of my spiritual explorations focus on Eastern mysticism, I will, from time to time, poke at the Abrahamic traditions. In doing so, I discovered a convergence between Jesus, Muhammad, and my preferred mystic, the Buddha.

All three of these mystics embarked on spiritual walkabouts—solitary journeys of contemplation, discovery, and self-inquiry: Jesus to the desert, Muhammad to the cave, Buddha across the plains of India. Furthermore, as part of these spiritual inquests, they all temporarily suspended their consumption of food.

Fasting is old. And while Christianity, Islam, and Buddhism don't always see eye to eye in terms of religious and political beliefs, their respective prophets—Jesus, Muhammed, and Buddha—were all dedicated fasters.

As Jesus confronted the devil, he was tempted neither by Satan's offerings nor evidently by lunch. This 40-day period of asceticism became known as Lent. Muhammad "intermittent fasted" on the regular and recommended time-restricted eating to all Muslims on the 13th, 14th, and 15th of every month.[1] These days of the lunar calendar are known as the "White Days" due to the full moon.[2] In fact, in Islam, fasting (*sawm*) is a requirement for attaining God-consciousness and one of the five pillars of the faith. Further, it is mythologized that Muhammed received the Koran during the ninth month of the Muslim calendar from the Angel Gabriel in a fasted state. The ninth month of the Islamic calendar is called Ramadan and one of its primary observances is fasting. Lastly, it is also said that the Buddha existed for a time, prior to his Bodhi tree revelation, on a single grain of rice daily.

Many religious traditions are built upon the notion that transcendence rests upon the perceived duality between spirit and body. We must eschew the corporeal for it is conjured from dust and to dust it will return. The body is ephemeral and subject to decay. It is susceptible to indulgences of the flesh, drink, and food. Hence, we lift ourselves up and out of our impermanence and into the eternal spiritual realm. We sublimate the appetite to grasp the infinite and find enlightenment.

But one need not be a follower of ancient scrolls to observe how cycles of fasting and eating are inherent to life's foundational fabric. The oppositional states of abundance and scarcity that foster balance between physiological growth and repair are part of human engineering.

Over hundreds of thousands of years, humans have evolved adaptively in relationship to these environmental prerogatives. For example, humans have developed genetic pathways that signal the body to store fat in anticipation of the impending winter, which serves as a naturally imposed sort of fast, a forced monasticism. Let me unpack this for a moment.

Long before we were stalking the Serengeti of Facebook, *Homo sapiens* foraged the savannah and forests for food. On a splendid fall afternoon in 10,327 B.C.E., Ffej stumbled to his great delight over a marvelous copse of barbary fig trees. The trees were so laden with ripe reddish teardrops that they appeared to be weeping.

Ffej enthusiastically harvested the figs, stuffing his satchel full to where its skin stretched. He proudly brought them back to his village, where the tribe gorged exuberantly on the figs until all that was left was a small mountain of stems and leaves in the center of the dining circle.

Ffej returned to the grove the following day with his men's group, who ransacked the remaining trees. They hauled a great bounty of figs back to the tribe, who devoured them with reckless abandon. After a week of great abundance, Ffej found his linen loin cloth to be a little tighter around his midsection. He didn't judge himself. His little paunch would come in handy soon enough as the scarcity of the upcoming winter loomed.

Food contains macro- and micronutrients that the body metabolizes for its myriad functions. Food is also a messenger. Certain constituents of food give signals to cells to act in certain ways. Let's focus for a moment on the molecular makeup of the fig and the directives that it delivers to the body. This exercise provides a window into the history of human evolutionary adaptations and how modern culture is upending them.

A medium-sized fig contains approximately 8 grams of sugar, 60 percent of which is glucose and the balance is fructose.[3] During digestion, these sugar carbohydrates are absorbed into the bloodstream.

Glucose triggers insulin from the pancreas almost like my daughters use Uber. Glucose hitches a ride from its insulin cabbie and gets taxied to the cell for the process of energy production. Fructose, on the other hand, doesn't have the insulin app on its iPhone and, instead, gets directly metabolized by the liver.

As the liver catabolizes fructose, chemical compounds called purines are released. The breakdown of purines produces uric acid which, in turn, signals your body's cells to become insulin resistant. When a cell develops insulin resistance, less glucose is able to enter it for the production of ATP and, instead, it remains in the bloodstream.

When glucose loiters in the blood for too long, it has numerous fates. Approximately 500 grams (depending on body mass) gets stored as glycogen in the liver as warehoused energy for a rainy day. Abandoned serum glucose can also form inflammatory glycoproteins, sometimes called advanced glycation end-products, by fusing with proteins like hemoglobin. Overwhelmingly, however, blood glucose is stored as triglycerides in adipocytes, commonly known as fat cells. In short, insulin resistance leads to fat accumulation. Take it from me.

It is theorized that 15 million years ago during the mid-Miocene ice age, the gene for uricase, the enzyme that breaks down uric acid, was silenced in our hominin ancestors.[4] This mutation was adaptive. As colder weather pervaded through Europe, it shortened the growing season and created longer periods of calorie paucity. Evolution stepped slowly in to address food scarcity by turning off the uricase gene, and, by extension, helping hominids become insulin resistant and warehouse fat.

This mechanism, resulting in fat storage, represents the brilliance of nature's intelligence. Across millennia, the body developed the adaptive mechanism of making Ffej a little fat during the abundant fall harvest because nature "knew" that the yang of the bright autumn yield would be dimmed by the yin of winter's fallow.

Ffej would require fat storage because food supplies naturally dwindle. Copious glucose would dry up. And, in order to produce the energy required for life, the body would need to break down triglycerides into free fatty acids and ketones, an alternate fuel source to glucose.

As Dr. Rich Johnson quips in his eponymously titled book, "Nature wants us to be fat."[5] Our bodies evolved to recognize fructose as a signal of upcoming scarcity and, in turn, store fat. But here's the problem: culture has now hijacked this evolutionary adaptation and rendered it maladaptive.

There is still considerable food scarcity in the world, and it is a salient problem that must be addressed as we hurtle into increasing climate volatility. However, most of the Western world suffers from overnutrition, not undernutrition. Significantly more people die from obesity and obesity-related diseases than from starvation.

Of course, the standard American diet is among the United States' most prominent exports so this phenomenon is hardly confined to the West. The overarching point is: Billions of people can now, on a whim, in the palm of their hand, or a short drive away avail themselves of any kind of food, in or out of season, on a 365-days per year, 7-days per week, 24-hours per day basis. This phenomenon represents one of our "biggest" Big MACs. Abundance is no longer balanced by scarcity. It's figs all day!

Well, if only it were. In reality, it is sugary drinks and snacks sweetened with high-fructose corn syrup all day . . . and all night: 84 percent of the items in the average grocery store contain added sugar—generally in the form of some unpronounceable fructose-based compound.[6] It's not just Coke, Oreos, and Skittles. It's salad dressings and pasta sauces, processed meats and potato chips, breakfast cereals, and baked goods—many of which are engineered in laboratories to hit your "bliss point" and trigger the neuropods in your gut to trick your brain into eating more.

The body, in response, is simply doing what it has evolved to do—store fat. The fact that 45 percent of Americans are obese is a predictable consequence of the body's adaptive mechanisms being hijacked by culture. What was once adaptive is now maladaptive.

Industrial farming and Big Food produce a glut of shelf-stable cheap ultra-processed calories designed to hijack the reward centers of your brain. The overconsumption of these "foods" directly contributes to the epidemics of the FUCKs: heart disease, cancer, diabetes, and neurodegenerative disease.

The disappearance of scarcity due to modern industrial agriculture and globalization gives our bodies a singular message: grow. And this monotone dispatch comes at the expense of repair.

The modern Western world tends to celebrate growth. Bigger is better is the motto of Western culture. But you don't want cancer to grow in your pancreas or fat to grow in your liver. You don't want beta-amyloid proteins to accumulate in your brain. And you don't want advanced glycation end-products to form in your bloodstream.

In order to counterbalance bulging bellies with cardio-metabolic health, many people (including yours truly) are consciously engineering scarcity in the form of intermittent fasting, also known as time-restricted eating. We're living a little bit more like Ffej.

Fasting can take on many forms from austere month-long water fasts to weekly 24-hour fasts to daily time-restricted eating to alternate day fasting. Any fasting protocol should be discussed with your primary care physician, particularly if you are pregnant, menstruating, or nursing. Regardless of which specific protocol you adopt, fasting should be integrated slowly to allow your body to acclimate to a new feeding schedule.

Fasting protocols were utilized in the 1920s for the treatment of epilepsy in children.[7] For reasons that still aren't completely clear, fasting appears to be neuroprotective and inhibits seizures. Of course, adherence to fasting protocols among children is not particularly reliable. Take it from a father of three daughters. This led doctors to develop fasting-mimicking diets, including the ketogenic diet, which, in some ways, mirrors the effects of fasting by keeping blood sugar and insulin levels low. This treatment for epilepsy drifted out of vogue as anticonvulsant drugs were developed. Still, fasting is considered a potent protocol for epilepsy as at least one-third of people suffering from seizures are resistant to medication.

Upon discovering I was diabetic, at the suggestion of Dr. Mark Hyman and Dr. Will Cole, I began intermittent fasting, ironically, but not purposefully, timed with Lent. Along with consolidating my food consumption into eight-hour blocks, I also affixed a continuous glucose monitor to my triceps. I then studied my blood sugar with a bookkeeper's zeal, and the results were amazing. In just four months, I brought down my fasting glucose levels from 125 mg/dL to 85 mg/dL. Time-restricted eating played a central role in this reversal of fortune.

The most extensive data on fasting relates to the 16-8 time-restricted eating protocol as researched by Satchin Panda's lab at the Salk Institute.[8] This is the protocol that I eased into to balance my unruly blood glucose levels.

My Fasting Regimen

Here is my daily fasting regime, and by no means am I neurotically fundamentalist about it. I consolidate all my eating in an eight-hour window between approximately 10:30 A.M. and 6:30 P.M. I take advantage of sleep as a de facto fasting period. Technically, the body is better at metabolizing food earlier in the day, so an earlier eating window might be more optimal, but I'd prefer to maintain some small semblance of a social life. It's become quite undemanding for me to abstain from food in the morning.

Thank God you can drink coffee or tea and maintain a fasted state, provided you don't add milk or sugars. And, indeed, I slurp an espresso, often with a shot of MCT oil about an hour after I wake up.

I drink plenty of lemon water. Lemons and limes are both effective glucose disposal agents. The acetic acid in vinegar is also a potent glucose sink, as are cinnamon and berberine, all of whom I have invited into my pantry.

Part of my morning ritual also includes a heaping tablespoon of green powder dumped in lukewarm water. I vigorously stir the pulverized nettle, barley grass, parsley, and basil leaf until my pint glass looks like a swamp sample. Don't forget the spirulina and chlorella or the kelp and nori. If the taste wasn't ghastly enough, I top it off with some liquified black pepper activated turmeric extract. I have estimated that this elixir of prebiotic fiber, phytonutrients, and adaptogens contains about 30 calories. I can burn that off in a few trips up and down my extensive outdoor staircase.

I combine intermittent fasting with a plant-focused ketogenic diet with occasional forays into omega-3-rich line-caught fish, some lean free-range chicken, and pasture-raised beef. I'll preserve a deep dive on diet for another book, but it is very related, specifically as it pertains to blood glucose levels. Everyone is different—but I can categorically claim that the overconsumption of refined sugar, refined grains, and ultra-processed meats is going to lead to high blood glucose levels (hyperglycemia), which is the precursor for type 2 diabetes and heart disease.

I am extremely intentional about how I break my fast and the cadence of different food types I consume. I focus on protein and fiber. The immediate consumption of carbohydrates at the end of a fast will get absorbed quickly into the bloodstream and spike glucose levels. The consumption of soluble fiber, on the contrary, will form a gel-like lattice in your small intestine and slow the absorption of food into your bloodstream. The consumption of protein—including all the nine essential amino acids—is crucial for myriad functions as well as being extremely satiating. I'll aim for 30 to 40 grams in the morning. A typical "break" fast might include three eggs, some leafy greens, two tablespoons of sauerkraut, and a generous slice of avocado. I might also go for plain non-fat Greek yogurt with some walnuts, flax, and sea salt.

To understand how fasting relates to your health, we need to dive into some of the mechanisms of metabolism. So, buckle your geek belt for a moment. I guarantee the more you understand the underlying functionality of your body, the more likely you are to adopt the protocols, tweak them, and get the results you're looking for.

So, here's a brief primer on metabolism and blood glucose. Your body needs energy to function. Fortunately, we all have our own energy-producing power plants called mitochondria. Every cell in our body, except our red blood cells, contains a different number of mitochondria that produce energy through a three-part process called cellular respiration. Your neurons, cardiac cells, "brown fat," and muscle cells boast the highest concentrations of mitochondria. This makes good sense given the energy requirements of your brain, heart, and muscles. More on brown fat later.

Your body employs glucose from dietary carbohydrates to generate energy in the form of ATP (adenosine triphosphate). Glucose is absorbed through your small intestine into the bloodstream and ushered into your cells by a peptide hormone called insulin, which is secreted from your pancreas. If you have too much serum glucose because you scarfed down a bucket of pasta with three Cokes, your pancreas will need to produce more insulin to fulfill its job. If this pattern continues, then eventually your cells become overwhelmed by the overabundant supply of glucose and shut its doors. In this scenario, you become insulin resistant.

As previously mentioned, when high levels of glucose are abandoned in the bloodstream, a few things can happen. Some glucose will get warehoused in the liver and muscle cells as glycogen. This glycogen gets released back into your bloodstream when you're running low on glucose. Additionally, serum glucose can "glycate" proteins like hemoglobin, the protein in your blood famously tasked with shepherding oxygen to your cells. These new glycoproteins are inflammatory and can increase the risk of vascular disease. Lastly, excess glucose is converted into triglycerides and stored in adipose tissue. This is why diabetes, which is reflected by recurring fasting glucose levels of 126 mg/dL and above, is so associated with obesity. Insulin is working overtime to vacate glucose from the bloodstream. In turn, the liver warehouses it as fat.

Through this basic understanding of metabolism, you can easily see how modern culture conspires to make us sick. The deadly combination of "breakfast any time" and an excess of refined carbohydrates leverages the body's adaptive mechanisms toward a sickly end.

Fasting lowers blood glucose levels, but, more importantly, it lowers insulin. Taking a break from stuffing my face reduced my blood sugar, which, in turn, gave my pancreas a much-needed pause. If the excess of insulin created a resistance to itself, then the absence of it produced a higher degree of sensitivity to it. My cells, specifically, the mitochondria in them, became more efficient at producing energy. This is why fasting was so central to upregulating my metabolic health and reversing my diabetes.

The benefits of fasting are multifarious and the practice activates a number of different processes in the body that I will now enumerate. Again, my primary focus is on 16-8 intermittent fasting, but I will touch upon other fasting protocols where appropriate. Of course, the time-restricted window imposed upon Ffej wasn't always predictable. Given the unreliability of food availability, Ffej mostly likely endured a variety of fasted states.

The Benefits

Fasting & Burning Fat

When you fast, blood glucose levels plummet. Low glucose levels trigger insulin's "yin" counterpart, a peptide hormone called glucagon. This hormone, also secreted from the pancreas, prompts a few processes, including:

1. The release of glycogen (stored glucose) from the liver
2. A process called gluconeogenesis (the endogenous production of glucose in the liver)
3. Lipolysis, the breakdown of triglycerides (fat) into free fatty acids (and glycerol) to produce energy

In other words, after about 12 to 18 hours, fasting triggers lipolysis, and your mitochondria begin to burn stored energy (a.k.a. fat) for energy instead of glucose. This state is also associated with ketosis in which free fatty acids become ketones that cells can leverage for energy production. Ketones have the additional benefit of reducing the production of free radicals and reactive oxygen species during energy production. I will expound more on free radicals later.

On a 36-hour water fast, given the dearth of available glucose and glycogen, the body will be in total fat-burning mode. Integrating a more severe fast once or twice a month can train the body to burn fat more readily and can improve the impacts of a 16-8 protocol.

Fasting & Weight Loss

For me, intermittent fasting was central to a tremendous amount of weight loss. I went from tipping the scales at 206 all the way down to 140, which was admittedly a bit below my ideal body weight.

One of the by-products of fasting *can* be weight loss but it's not guaranteed. It obviously depends on the amount and quality of the food you eat during the feeding window. You can eat eight pints of Chubby Hubby, a Ben & Jerry's favorite, within eight hours. That doesn't end well. However, generally, one tends to constrict calories (and consume the "right" calories) when one is focusing close attention on a behavior like fasting. There is a phenomenon called the Hawthorne effect, where individuals modify or improve an aspect of their behavior in response to their awareness of being observed. Fasting is a form of self-observation and tends to result in adaptive behavior change.

Further, there are studies in mice that suggest you can eat the EXACT same diet and maintain your weight in a 24-hour feeding cycle or *lose* weight in a time-restricted protocol. In other words, the same amount of nutrition and calories will have a more adaptive impact if consumed in a restricted window.

For the vain among us, weight loss can obviously help you look "better." But losing weight in the form of visceral fat has more profound benefits. The oxidation of adipose tissue lessens the workload on the heart and reduces inflammation. I will extrapolate on this mechanism in the resistance training section.

Fasting & Cellular Cleanup

Fasting is a signal that activates a cellular pathway known as AMPK (AMP-activated protein kinase). In low-energy "fasted" states,

AMPK opposes mTOR (mammalian target of rapamycin), the pathway for cellular growth. I explore these pathways in greater detail at the end of this chapter. This inhibition of mTOR triggers autophagy—the body's system for cleaning out dysfunctional proteins known as senescent cells. *Auto* means "self" and *phagy* is Latin for "eat." So, according to its literal translation, autophagy is a form of the body "eating itself." It involves the formation of a double-membraned vesicle called an autophagosome, which engulfs the cellular components to be degraded. The autophagosome then fuses with a lysosome, creating an autolysosome where the contents are degraded.

This process enables damaged proteins to be broken down into their amino acid building blocks so that they can then be upcycled by your cells for new protein synthesis. The housekeeping process is a crucial cellular process for longevity.

There is some debate about how long the body must be fasted to trigger autophagy. Most doctors and experts believe that the body doesn't enter autophagy until it has been fasted for 24 hours. However, the overarching point is that the imposition of deliberate food scarcity allows the body to rest and repair.

Fasting & Mitochondria

Humans need energy to live. Full stop. And our ability to make energy depends completely on the jelly bean–shaped organelles inside our cells known as mitochondria. These organelles are responsible for taking energy substrates like glucose and fat and transmuting them into energy currency.

Mitochondrial activity declines with age, but AMPK activation counteracts this deterioration by triggering mitochondrial biogenesis, the production of new, healthy mitochondria. In this way, fasting helps to build new energy factories in your cells.

Having greater numbers of optimally functioning mitochondria is awfully important as when we stop producing energy, we die.

Fasting & DNA Expression

Every cell in your body contains DNA, which has a fixed nucleotide sequence that is unique to you. Your DNA "expresses" itself by giving protein recipes to RNA, which ventures out of the cell nucleus into the cytoplasm and delivers these transcriptions to your ribosomes that, in turn, produce proteins. While your DNA is fixed, its expression is not. Your *epigenome* marks your DNA in a manner that influences the timing and content of its recipes. To reiterate a musical analogy from Part I, your DNA are the piano keys, your epigenome is the piano player.

Fasting activates sirtuins, a family of seven proteins that regulate cellular function and gene expression. Sirtuins are virtuoso pianists in that they help to maintain proper genomic expression. They also upgrade mitochondrial function and suppress tumor growth. The Australian biologist David Sinclair famously demonstrated that depriving yeast and mice of calories significantly extended their lifespan through the activation of sirtuin pathways.[9] To be clear, I am neither a single-celled organism or a rodent, and it remains unclear if sirtuin activation will have much impact on my lifespan, but it is compelling to consider.

Parenthetically, eating plants rich in polyphenols, like resveratrol, may also activate sirtuins and, not surprisingly, the plants that are highest in these phytonutrients are the most "stressed" ones. Plants, like humans, can positively respond to low-grade stressors (like drought) and generate self-protecting compounds. Grapes used for the production of wine are often purposefully stressed by vintners. Hence, wine (particularly pinot noir) contains resveratrol (but not nearly enough to have any significant impact). One can supplement with resveratrol (and NMN—the precursor to NAD+) to stimulate sirtuin activity. I cover this topic in greater depth in Chapter 18, "Eating Stressed Plants."

Fasting & the Microbiome

In your large intestine, there are 39 trillion bacteria that mediate a wide variety of physiological systems from digestion to immunity to mood regulation. These bugs are separated from your bloodstream (and most of your immune system) by a microscopically thin epithelial wall. The breakdown of the integrity of the tight junctions that make up this wall is called intestinal permeability (leaky gut!).

When your gut is leaky, endotoxins seep into your bloodstream, eliciting an inflammatory response. If dysbiosis (disruption of the gut microbiome) and permeability persist, you can end up with chronic inflammation. Your body can also begin attacking itself. Autoimmune diseases such as ulcerative colitis, intestinal bowel disease, and Crohn's disease are increasingly common due to poor gut health.

Research into the impacts of fasting on the microbiome is still preliminary. However, there is some early data that demonstrates that 16-8 time-restricted feeding can lead to an increase in *Akkermansia*, a beneficial bacterial strain, as well as an uptick in the production of butyrate, a short-chain fatty acid produced by bacteria that promotes epithelial integrity and upregulates insulin sensitivity.[10]

However, long-term fasts can have the opposite impact. Extended fasting can alter the composition of the gut microbiota. Some bacteria may diminish due to a lack of nutrients, while others might turn to the mucosal lining as a source of energy, potentially leading to mucosal degradation. This shift in microbial populations can affect the integrity of the gut barrier, increasing the risk of issues like increased intestinal permeability, which can allow toxins and pathogens to enter the bloodstream.

If you're going to engage in longer fasts, then it is important to rebuild your gut flora when the fast is completed. You can do this through the consumption of fermented foods and with certain high-quality probiotic supplements.

The Psychology of Fasting

In summary, fasting improves metabolic function and addresses many of the hallmarks of aging. It was essential to my metabolic health journey. I lost weight and burned fat. Because I stopped eating at 7 P.M., my sleep benefited as I drifted into dreamland with my food digested.

However, while I can identify many of the physiological attributes of fasting, the most potent benefits may be psychological.

In many respects, fasting became a spiritual pursuit. When I started the 16-8 protocol, I had a craving not to crave. (Of course, this is a paradox.) Still, I didn't want to incessantly pine for late-night trips to Denny's as a means for comfort. I wanted to eschew the pursuit of external agents to satiate my internal needs. But there was more.

Just because I consolidated my eating into eight hours didn't mean I didn't get hungry during the other 16. However, my "discipleship" to my practice prohibited me from mindlessly wandering to the cupboard for salt and vinegar chips. I was forced to stop and witness the hunger.

The brilliant writer and Holocaust survivor Viktor Frankl famously wrote, "Between stimulus and response, there is a space. In that space is our power to choose our response. In our response lies our growth and our freedom." In the space between the stimulus of hunger and the response of eating, I began to observe the nature of the hunger and ask myself, "Is this hunger a biological need or an emotional desire?"

So often, in this space, I discovered that I was eating my feelings. My trips to the pantry assuaged my boredom or anxiety or some insult thrown at me on Instagram. Fasting helped me make unconscious behavior conscious. It helped me to delineate between needs and desires.

This skill began to punctuate my life in areas that I didn't expect.

I realized that if I could stop capriciously craving food, then I could certainly stop instinctively grabbing for my phone or the wine bottle or the credit card in search of ephemeral pleasure. When my children misbehaved, instead of reacting, I could find the space to examine the origin of their behavior and respond appropriately.

The practice of fasting, I learned, is applicable well beyond food. It's Good Stress—short-term discomfort in exchange for long-term real comfort.

As the Buddha instructed, the cessation of craving is a stepping stone to nirvana, to liberation, and to contentment.

Fasting Protocols

Here I outline some general protocols for fasting. Of course, everyone is different, so you will want to experiment to find the right regimen that suits your bio-individuality.

- You always want to wait at least one hour after you wake up before eating.
- You ideally want three full hours of digestion prior to sleep. Sleep, of course, is a nonfeeding period, but just because you are not eating doesn't mean your body has gone into a fasted state. If you ate a huge meal an hour ago, your body is still spending considerable energy digesting and metabolizing food.
- The ideal feeding window is earlier in the day as your body is more optimized to metabolize macronutrients, particularly protein, earlier in the day. That said, a 9 A.M. to 5 P.M. feeding window is not particularly friendly. Find the schedule that works for you.
- Start slow. Phase in a fasting protocol. While the preponderance of data supports a 16-8 protocol, there is also research to suggest that a 12-12 protocol can also be effective.
- Try to be relatively consistent with your feeding window. If it's 10 to 6, then try to maintain that schedule without getting obsessive.
- When breaking a fast, focus on eating fiber, protein, and healthy fats. For example, you might break a fast with plain Greek yogurt and walnuts. Or, you might opt for an egg with avocado, sauerkraut, or spinach. You want to avoid sugar and "naked" carbs. Consuming fiber and protein and eschewing sugars and starches will keep blood glucose levels in check.
- Experiment with a 24- or 36-hour fast once a month.
- Always consult your doctor prior to starting a fasting protocol, particularly if you're pregnant, breastfeeding, or menstruating. As an additional resource, Dr. Mindy Pelz has an excellent book about fasting for women titled *Fast Like a Girl*.

- Lastly, avoid being neurotic about fasting. There is a condition that is growing in prevalence called orthorexia in which people become obsessive with healthy eating and associated restrictive behaviors. A fanatical attempt to attain optimal health through attention to diet can end up leading to malnourishment, loss of relationships, and poor quality of life.

THE BODY IN BALANCE

At the end of every chapter of the Good Stress protocols in Part II, I will include a section titled "The Body in Balance." This segment will explore the oppositional molecules, pathways, and processes that are brought into balance by the Good Stress protocol featured in the chapter.

I maintain that understanding the mechanisms behind the protocols makes you more likely to adopt them. Further, with a foundational understanding of the body's functionality, you can better tweak the protocols to meet your needs. These sections will, at times, revisit the information imparted in the preceding chapter but through a different, more scientific lens.

I toyed with titling the section "For Geeks Only," but that seemed exclusionary. And, really, anyone can understand these concepts. Just look at me. Only four years ago, I didn't understand 90 percent of this science. But, slowly, like a child learning to play "Chopsticks" on the piano, I became more fluent. You can too.

Growth vs. Repair

Fostering balance between growth and repair may be the most critical area of focus for optimal well-being, both in the human body and in society at large.

The modern world sanctifies growth in virtually every aspect. The yang overshadows the yin in the West—and now also in much of the East. Bigger is better. Corporations yearn for "hockey stick" revenue growth. Gargantuan McMansions are a badge of success. Megafarms dominate industrial agriculture. Like hungry ghosts, we fill our massive tanks with fossil fuels such that 6,000-pound SUVs can haul around 180 pounds of human flesh and bone.

The metrics by which we measure societal success are almost always anchored in expansion. Economists tout the year-over-year growth of the GDP, the S&P 500, and the Dow Jones Industrial Average. But, of course, these numbers rarely mirror the true underlying health of a society. They don't account for how a society repairs its land, its infrastructure, and its relationships with past transgressions.

Like a healthy society, a healthy human being is a balance of growth and repair with both processes transpiring at the right times. There are a lot of terms and processes that relate to growth and repair in the human organism. We will explore some here.

Anabolism vs. Catabolism

Anabolism and catabolism are two opposing metabolic processes that occur within cells and organisms. You can think of them as construction and destruction. You build things up. And you break things down. The two together are tango partners in the larger dance we call metabolism.

Anabolic processes refer to the fabricating of complex molecules from simpler ones, typically requiring energy input. For example, muscle hypertrophy and bone development are anabolic.

Anabolic processes include protein synthesis, the formation of glycogen from glucose and the synthesis of fatty acids.

Catabolic processes, on the other hand, refer to the breaking down of complex molecules into simpler ones, releasing energy in the process. Examples of catabolic processes include the breakdown of glucose through cellular respiration, fatty acids for energy, and proteins into amino acids.

These two processes are interconnected and work in harmony to maintain the energy balance within the body. Together, they ensure that the body has the necessary building blocks and energy to carry out its various functions.

Growth: Mitosis, Hypertrophy & Hyperplasia

You're a bit flaky. Literally. You lose 40,000 dead skin cells each minute or about 2,000 during the time that it took to read this sentence. This amounts to about 50 million skin cell funerals every day. So why aren't your insides overflowing out onto the floor?

Mitosis is a process of cell division that results in the production of two identical daughter cells. I have three daughters by other means. Skin cells, along with blood and muscle cells, are replaced through mitosis, keeping your guts thankfully on the inside and protecting it from pathogens. Mitosis is a fundamental process for the growth of tissues in multicellular organisms in which the genetic material of a cell is replicated and separated into two cells.

Hypertrophy is the goal of curls, squats, and bench presses. It is the process of increasing the breadth of tissues and organs by enlarging the size of their constituent cells. This can occur in response to various stimuli, such as exercise or weightlifting, which causes the muscle cells to increase in size in order to handle the increased workload.

Hyperplasia is a different type of growth. Instead of increasing the size of the cell, the process of hyperplasia increases the number of cells in a tissue or organ, resulting in an overall increase in size. This can occur in response to various stimuli, such as hormonal changes, growth factors, or chronic irritation.

There are two types of hyperplasia: physiological and pathological. Physiological hyperplasia occurs in response to normal physiological processes, such as during embryonic development, tissue regeneration after injury, or during the menstrual cycle. Pathological hyperplasia, on the other hand, occurs as a result of abnormal or excessive growth signals and can be a precursor to cancer.

Repair: Apoptosis & Autophagy

Apoptosis, also known as programmed cell death, is a process by which cells intentionally die off in order to maintain the overall health of an organism. This process would be very useful in politics but, alas, it is confined to the human body and unavailable to the body politic.

Apoptosis is a natural process that helps remove damaged, infected, or unwanted cells, preventing them from causing harm to the body. Apoptosis can be triggered by a variety of factors, including cellular stress, DNA damage, and signaling molecules.

Autophagy technically means self-eating, wonderful at the cellular level but not otherwise recommended. It's best categorized as the body's recycling program. It involves the formation of autophagosomes, double-membraned vesicles that engulf damaged cellular components, and the subsequent breakdown of these components by lysosomes, enzyme-laden cellular organelles. Autophagy disassembles damaged proteins into their component amino acid building blocks that the body can then upcycle into new proteins.

Autophagy can be activated by various stimuli, such as nutrient deprivation, fasting, exercise, and by the consumption of specific foods and compounds like green tea, turmeric, coffee, ginger, reishi mushrooms, and broccoli sprouts.

AMPK vs. mTOR: The Yin-Yang Pathways

AMPK (AMP-activated protein kinase) and mTOR (mammalian target of rapamycin) are two interlinked and opposing cellular pathways involved in sensing the availability of nutrients and energy and regulation of cell growth.

AMPK is our yin. It is activated by a decrease in energy (ATP) sometimes induced by fasting or exercise, and it inhibits cell growth. AMPK activates autophagy, the breakdown of dysfunctional cells previously described. AMPK promotes catabolic processes such as fatty acid oxidation (the breaking down of fats for use in energy production).

MTOR is our yang. MTOR is activated by growth factors such as insulin and amino acids. Insulin and insulin growth factor (IGF-1) is a response to glucose consumption (i.e., eating carbohydrates). The presence of insulin subsequently triggers mTOR, which promotes cell growth, protein synthesis, and cell proliferation.

As we have discussed, the human body is a dynamic interplay of opposing forces. The key to health is fostering a balance between growth and repair, activity and restoration, and construction and destruction. Anabolic processes are wonderful when you're growing muscle cells for bulging biceps but highly undesirable when you're growing tumor cells in breast tissue.

As a general observation, too many of us are experiencing overgrowth or the dysregulation of mTOR signaling, which is linked to cancer and diabetes. This phenomenon stems from an excessive emphasis on consumption, growth, and expansion at the expense of rest and conservation. Similarly, the activation of AMPK, which has been associated with improved metabolic health and increased lifespan, is a reminder of the importance of restoration and balance in maintaining cellular health and vitality.

Just as nature promises a spring with every winter, our bodies are naturally programmed for periods of restoration and regrowth. We simply need to align with nature's course. This sometimes means simulating the environment in which our bodies evolved and imposing the "yin" qualities of repair such as scarcity and darkness.

Insulin vs. Glucagon

Balancing blood sugar levels is essential to health. It's central to energy production. When we stop making energy, we cross into the afterlife.

When we talk about blood sugar, we're specifically referring to glucose. The chemical formula for glucose is $C_6H_{12}O_6$. It is arguably a hydrocarbon, like oil or coal. And your mitochondria are a combustion engine transmuting this molecule into energy and releasing carbon dioxide and water. This process is called cellular respiration.

Glucose is a critical molecule. However, when it's chronically overabundant in the bloodstream, it can get converted to triglycerides and stored in fat cells. Too much serum glucose leads to type 2 diabetes, which can cause neuropathy, vision loss, kidney disease, dementia, and cardiovascular disease.

Glucose management relies on a peptide hormone known as insulin. Insulin is among the body's master hormones. Insulin is made by the pancreas and chauffeurs glucose entering the bloodstream from the small intestine to cells for energy production. Insulin has other subsidiary roles as well relating to the breakdown of protein and lipids and uptake of amino acids and potassium, but its primary job is to deliver glucose to the cells. This task is compromised when the cells don't want any more glucose. Too much glucose delivery to the cells is akin to too many raw materials arriving at a factory. Production cannot keep up with the quantity of parts. Central receiving gets overwhelmed when the supply chain is too heavy and eventually closes its doors. When a cell closes its doors to glucose, it is a condition known as insulin resistance.

Spurred by the cells, glucose acts like a jilted lover and causes all types of havoc in the bloodstream.

While insulin receives most of the headlines in the *Hormone Gazette*, it has a rarely celebrated counterpart: glucagon.

Glucagon is also a peptide hormone produced in the pancreas. While insulin is produced to keep blood glucose from rising too high, glucagon keeps blood glucose from dropping too low. These two hormones ideally collaborate in the hopes of avoiding both hyperglycemia (blood sugar levels that are too high) and hypoglycemia (blood sugar levels that are too low).

When blood sugar levels drop, the pancreas releases glucagon, which signals the liver to do a number of things in order to preserve raw materials for energy production. You can't stop making energy or you die.

Glucagon tells the liver to release glycogen (stockpiled glucose). It also messages the liver to make glucose from amino acids and glycerol in a process called gluconeogenesis. Lastly, it triggers the process of lipolysis in which triglycerides are broken down into fatty acids and glycerol. These fatty acids, also known as ketone bodies, are used by the cells to produce energy (instead of using glucose). This state is known as ketosis and has been associated with the ketogenic diet, which is low in sugar and carbohydrate consumption.

When the body is fed the proper nutrients (not too much refined sugar, refined grains, and ultra-processed foodstuffs), then insulin and glucagon cooperate to produce little crests and troughs of glucose levels. It is perfectly healthy to have moderate postprandial (after eating) increases in blood sugar. However, you want your levels to look like the rolling hills of Georgia and not the peaks and valleys of the Colorado Rockies. Health is in the middle, in the Goldilocks zone.

CHAPTER 11

THE DRYING OF THE SHEETS

Deliberate Cold Therapy

The bourgeois prefers comfort to pleasure, convenience to liberty, and a pleasant temperature to the deathly inner consuming fire.

— Herman Hesse

Candidly and simply, I abhor the cold. Submerging myself in an ice bath is among the most ghastly activities I could name. However, I was pleased to discover that I was not alone. Even the "Iceman," Wim Hof, prefers a balmy tropical day to a frigid one. Wim and his extensive, fun-loving brood visited Commune Topanga for three wonderful weeks in March 2019.

When I asked him where he prefers to holiday, he replied, "Anywhere with a palm tree!"

"Not the cold?" I asked, surprised.

"I hate the cold!" Wim thundered like a Norse god. And then belly laughed, shaking the ground around us.

For 21 glorious days, we had a commercial ice delivery at dawn and a wine delivery at dusk. The anti-inflammatory attributes of the ice plunge came in handy in more ways than one. Beyond the many other virtues of cold therapy that I will extoll in this chapter, I will say that nothing cures a hangover like immersing into a 40-degree bath.

Wim's visit was marvelous. Every morning, amid the thick marine layer, I would watch him toodle out naked to the plunge and sink in with utter ease. The temperature of the water hovered just above freezing. Ice blocks bobbed like apples on water's upper crust. Unmoved, Wim would rest there like a Buddha, with just an intimation of a smile across his face. After fifteen minutes, he'd rouse himself from the ice, don a miniscule pair of shorts, and go tend the garden. I would join him there.

Upon noticing me, Wim would launch immediately into a diatribe on the health benefits of breathwork and ice bath immersion with the same vim and vigor as he had the previous day. He bellowed on about the science, selling it to me as if he'd never met me. This pattern repeated itself throughout his stay. Part of Wim's remarkable success rests on his indefatigable enthusiasm for this singular practice. He's like Taylor Swift on tour. He plays the hits. And people love it.

Every afternoon, plungers of all ilks drifted into Commune. Wim held court like a king, leading the brave goose-bumped masses in super-ventilating breathwork, ice bathing, and his patented horse dance.

I had assiduously avoided cold water all my life. The mere sight of a freshwater lake was enough to palpate my heart until I was baptized by Wim Hof himself. Wim did the impossible. He got me into the ice. And this most dreaded ritual became one of the most important components of my health journey.

One of the reasons Ffej Onsark didn't feel separate from nature was his proximity to it. Nature was quite literally his home. Unlike our suburban boxes, Ffej's small hut of branches and grass had no digital thermostat on the wall. Hence, he had no ability to control the ambient temperature. He was subject to the weather fluctuations of the high desert, which might be alternately scorching on a summer's day and frigid on a winter's night. Ffej was not unduly bothered by nature's vacillations because his body was equipped with an analog internal thermostat located just above the roof of his mouth and below his nose.

The preoptic area of the frontal cortex in concert with the hypothalamus regulates core body temperature based on skin temperature. Because the skin is more exposed to the environment, skin temperature fluctuates more widely than core temperature. Normal skin temperature for healthy adults ranges between 92.3 and 98.4 Fahrenheit (or 33–37 degrees Celsius), lower than the 98.6 degrees Fahrenheit average core temperature. When we're feeling a bit off and "take our temperature," we are attempting to measure our core temperature, which is why taking a rectal measurement is the most reliable, if somewhat awkward, method to obtain an accurate value.

We have long been taught that a normal core temperature is 98.6 degrees. But, surprise, there is nothing stable about your organism. It is in constant flux. Core temperature naturally fluctuates with your circadian rhythm, varying from 97.7–99.5 degrees Fahrenheit over the course of the day.

Your core body temperature peaks in the late afternoon and then slowly decreases. This decline in core temperature plays a key role in your ability to fall asleep. Your body temperature usually reaches its nadir around 4:00 A.M. and then slowly rises. Crests and troughs—such is the nature of nature.

Normal fluctuations in ambient temperature Ffej experienced led to the development of adaptive mechanisms that resulted in greater resilience, reduced inflammation, upregulated metabolic function, better circulation, improved energy and alertness, increased stress management skills, and reduced muscle soreness.

Unlike Ffej, I can set my *external* thermostat, the one affixed to the wall in the den, to maintain a snug ambience of 72 degrees irrespective of vacillations in weather patterns. I owe Warren Johnson a debt for this luxury. He invented the thermostat in 1883 to minimize disruption in his classroom. The modern air conditioner was invented 19 years later by Willis Haviland Carrier in 1902. Carrier designed the first modern air-conditioning system to control the humidity and temperature in a printing plant, improving the quality and consistency of the printed paper. Honeywell debuted the first digital thermostat in the 1980s and, of course, now we can manipulate ambient temperature from myriad phone applications.

These innovations might satisfy my psychological desire for comfort, but they make poor use of my hard-earned biological advantages. They allow me to linger listlessly in thermoneutrality, the state of the environment where the ambient temperature is such that the body does not need to expend extra energy to maintain its core temperature.

Long-term exposure to thermoneutral conditions leads to a decrease in basal metabolic rate. This is because the body's thermoregulatory mechanisms (like shivering or sweating) that help burn calories are less active. Over time, this can contribute to metabolic inefficiency. Furthermore, regular exposure to non-thermoneutral conditions (both cold and hot) can enhance the body's ability to adapt to varying temperatures, a concept known as thermal adaptation. Living constantly in thermoneutral conditions diminishes this adaptive capacity, making sudden temperature changes more challenging to cope with.

As I will elucidate, deliberate cold exposure through ice plunges and cold showers serve to realign us with health-conferring adaptive mechanisms. As with many ancient protocols, before we had an empirical understanding of cold therapy, its benefits were intuited and cultivated by the sages of the East.

The Drying of the Sheets

In 1981, Herbert Benson, a cardiologist at Harvard Medical School, set out to study the ancient meditation practices of Tibetan Buddhist monks. With the Dalai Lama's blessing, Benson spent roughly a decade in remote regions of the Himalayas in northern India researching an especially intense technique known as Tummo, or inner heat practice.

Benson witnessed monks wrapped in 3-by-6-foot cotton sheets that had been soaked in 49-degree water. To add further insult to injury, the monks were made to sit quietly in a room no warmer than 40 degrees Fahrenheit. Leveraging a yoga technique known as Tummo, they entered a state of deep meditation. The Tummo practice combines yogic postures, breath control, and complex visualizations that create an internal energy such that "psychic heat" becomes real heat. The breathing, known as vase breathing, involves slowly inhaling and then holding the breath with a swallow, which creates intra-abdominal pressure that bulges the belly—hence the name *vase* because the belly looks like a vase. During the breath hold, the yogi pulls upward from his perineum and pushes downward from his throat, creating a kind of internal pressure chamber. All the while the complicated visualization is performed. This is repeated many times over in a single meditation session.

For untrained people, the frigid sheets and environment would produce uncontrollable shivering. If body temperatures continue to drop under these conditions, the result can be severe hypothermia and even death. However, 30 minutes after the monks began their Tummo practice, steam began rising from their sheets. As a result of body heat produced by the monks during meditation, the sheets dried in about an hour. Attendants removed the sheets, then covered the meditators with a second chilled, wet wrapping. Each monk was required to dry three sheets over a period of several hours.

The underlying purpose of the Tummo is not to turn monks into a clothes dryer, but rather to create a psychic blaze that rises in the body's central energetic channel. This internal heat is meant to incinerate the mental habits of jealousy, pride, and anger, resulting in heightened levels of joy and a nondual state of absolute clarity. In other words, the purpose is enlightenment; dry sheets are just the consequence.

The historical use of deliberate cold therapy hasn't been applied exclusively to robed meditators. It has also been leveraged as a technique to train the military.

The United States Navy's Sea, Air, and Land Teams, commonly known as the Navy SEALs, are the U.S. Navy's primary special operations force and a component of the Naval Special Warfare Command. Navy SEALs are renowned for their physical fitness, mental toughness, and exceptional ability to perform complex missions under highly stressful conditions. Navy SEALs train extensively in cold-water environments using a method known as cold-water conditioning. The training is designed to build their physical and mental resilience.

Surf torture is one of the most notorious parts of Navy SEALs training. In this exercise, trainees link arms and wade into the ocean until they are waist or chest deep, and then they lie down in the surf. They must remain there for extended periods of time, sometimes in the middle of the night, which quickly leads to onset of hypothermia.

Trainees must rely on mental toughness and team camaraderie to endure this challenge. Other unfathomable drills include swimming long distances in cold water and bobbing up and down in cold water—often with hands and feet bound.

While I would never recommend either Navy SEAL training or drenching yourself in icy bedsheets, there are clear psychological and physiological health benefits associated with deliberate cold therapy.

The preponderance of data focuses around ice baths in which your body, up to your neck, is fully submerged in cold water. How cold? It depends. Cold and its accompanying discomfiture is highly subjective and relative. Evidence suggests that benefits can be conferred through exposure to water with a temperature as high as 60 degrees Fahrenheit (about 15 degrees Celsius). Other hard-core plungers prefer a bath closer to a frosty 40 degrees.

To obtain the health-conferring results, the water must simply *feel* uncomfortable. And, of course, this practice requires caution. Hypothermia is no laughing matter. So, the trick is to ease into it. Data suggests that four sessions per week totaling cumulative 11 minutes of exposure will confer benefits. If you don't have access to a cold plunge, cold showers are an acceptable alternative. There's simply less data on cold showers because it's harder to conduct experiments with showers as the conditions are less controllable.

The Benefits

Surely you've seen star athletes like Novak Djokovic or LeBron James soaking in giant tubs of ice. Why make oneself so miserable? Well, you've probably sprained your ankle once or twice, so you know at least one answer.

One of the primary benefits of cold therapy is the reduction of inflammation. The cold can constrict blood vessels and reduce swelling. Many athletes use cold-water immersion to speed up recovery after intense training sessions or physical performances. Again, the cold helps alleviate muscle soreness and inflammation. But the benefits of deliberate cold-water therapy run much deeper than treating inflammation.

Mental Resilience

Sudden immersion in cold water can initiate a series of responses in your body that may result in discomfort or even a sense of panic. When you enter very cold water, your body first experiences a cold-shock response. This is an involuntary response characterized by an uncontrollable gasp for air and increased respiratory rate, heart rate, and blood pressure. Levels of adrenaline can increase 500 percent. This reaction can create a sense of panic.

These are normal adaptive bottom-up responses of the sympathetic nervous system. However, as they pass, then there is a moment—a space—to leverage your breath and your neo-mammalian prefrontal cortex. You apply top-down voluntary pressure on to bottom-up involuntary response. Through mental concentration and use of the breath, you can neutralize feelings of panic. This practice becomes a protean skill. You build psychological resilience that spills over into your life such that you can manage stress as it inevitably arises.

The key is to start deliberate cold therapy gradually and then increase durations of exposure and decrease temperature over time. By breaking through "walls" of discomfort, as Andrew Huberman puts it, you will build the capacity to think clearly and react appropriately under stress. This is useful in traffic as well as in more life-or-death situations. In short, doing hard things makes doing other hard things easier.

Mood Regulation

The significant elevation in adrenaline is certainly going to make you alert. Hence, cold-water therapy is an excellent protocol for any activity that benefits from alertness—like learning. Cold therapy sharpens mental acuity and focus and can be a powerful tool for neuroplasticity. If I have a late-night drive ahead of me, a cold shower will ensure that I am attentive. Cold-water therapy appears to raise adrenaline without significantly elevating cortisol. Hence, you can experience alertness without feeling stress.

A study conducted at Charles University in the Czech Republic found that cold-water immersion at 57.2 degrees Fahrenheit lowered rectal temperature and increased metabolic rate by 350 percent. Cortisol concentrations tended to decrease, while plasma noradrenaline and dopamine concentrations were increased by 530 percent and by 250 percent respectively.[1]

Dopamine is a powerful mood regulator providing a feeling of reward and motivation. Cold-water therapy upregulates dopamine release over a protracted period of time, not just during the session.[2] You may experience 48 hours of elevated dopamine levels post-cold immersion.[3]

In this manner, cold therapy may be a powerful treatment for addiction as it stimulates the same dopamine receptors as drugs without the detrimental long-term impacts.

Cold & Metabolic Health

When you immerse yourself into an ice bath or cold shower, your core body temperature will plummet. As described, your body is equipped with an internal thermostat that maintains a core body temperature in the Goldilocks zone, around 98.6 degrees Fahrenheit (37 Celsius). When your temperature drops, your body springs into action in a process called thermogenesis. Your body needs to burn energy to generate heat to re-establish homeostasis.

Much of this activity is carried out in a specific type of tissue known as brown fat. Brown fat is rich in mitochondria and serves as the body's furnace, upregulating core temperature through energy production when the body gets cold. Triggering thermogenesis in your brown fat can actually "beige" your "white fat." More on the roles of white fat in a few pages (pun intended). Further, cold showers and ice baths can lead to mitobiogenesis, the creation of new mitochondria, in your white fat.

Stacking Fasting & Cold Therapy

Of course, your mitochondria need a fuel source to create heat. If you are in a fasted state and/or have a low-glycemic diet, there is very little glucose around to burn. In this case, your body will require another energy substrate and will have very little choice but to convert triglycerides to free fatty acids and ketones for fuel. The combination of fasting and cold-water therapy can be a powerful way to oxidize fat and lose weight. This protocol "stack" is most effective if you expose yourself to cold before eating your first bite of the day.

When I started cold plunging before breaking my fast around 10:30 A.M., you could almost witness the fat burning off. According to metabolic scientist Dr. Susanna Søeberg, you can maximize this impact by refusing a towel and letting yourself shiver. Don't huddle; just let yourself air dry. Yeah . . . brrrrr.

Protocol

Deliberate cold therapy can be accomplished in a number of ways. As I previously mentioned, the preponderance of data focuses around ice baths in which your body, up to your neck, is fully submerged in cold water.

But not everyone has access to a cold plunge. Of course, you can use your bathtub as a facsimile and fill it with cold water, adding ice. The simplest and most accessible way to avail yourself of cold therapy is to take a cold shower. You can start your cold-therapy protocol gradually by simply ending your shower cold.

The temperature of the water is extremely subjective and bio-individual. The benefits can be conferred even at 60 degrees, provided that the water feels uncomfortably cold. Other hard-core plungers prefer a bath closer to a frosty 40 degrees.

Data suggests that four sessions per week totaling 11 minutes of exposure will confer the benefits I have enumerated.[4]

If you're in it for the metabolic benefits, try not to dry off. And consider timing your cold therapy with your fasting protocol and take your cold medicine prior to eating your first bite of food.

Of course, these protocols must be safely administered and under consultation with your doctor. Hypothermia is no joke. And, in very rare cases, cold shock can cause heart attack due to severe vasoconstriction. As noted, cold is extremely subjective. All that's required is that it *feel* uncomfortable. So, start slow and gradually progress to colder temperatures and longer durations.

THE BODY IN BALANCE

White Fat vs. Brown Fat

The word *fat* is plump with meanings.

To begin with, there are a multitude of dietary fats that you consume. Fats, like carbohydrates, consist mainly of carbon, hydrogen, and oxygen. They are sometimes referred to as long-chain carbon molecules because they are constituted from long chains of carbon atoms that are bonded together.

There are saturated fats named thusly because they are "saturated" with hydrogen molecules. They are most often found in animal-based foods like beef, pork, poultry, full-fat dairy products, eggs, and tropical oils. These fats distinguish themselves as being solid at room temperature.

Monounsaturated fats are liquid at room temperature but start to harden when chilled. There is a high concentration of monounsaturated fats in olive oil, avocadoes, various seeds (including pumpkin and sunflower), pecans, almonds, and peanuts.

Then there are the polyunsaturated fats (PUFAs), including anti-inflammatory omega-3s found in fatty fish, chia, flax, and some algae and pro-inflammatory omega-6s located in some nuts, seeds, eggs, and vegetable oils.

To be clear, foods have different concentrations of various fat types. For example, most of an egg's total fatty acid composition is monounsaturated (approximately 38 percent), 16 percent is polyunsaturated, and only 28 percent is saturated.

Lastly, there are the odious trans fats which, chemically, more closely resemble plastic than they do other fats or oils. These should be avoided at all costs.

Dietary fat hired a terrible branding agency. It is only logical to think that consuming fats would make you fat (and then give you heart disease). Indeed, we thought that was the case for decades. However, that theory has been disproven—sort of. Dietary fat *is* highly caloric and will get stored as fat if consumption outstrips energy burn. The overconsumption of saturated fat can, in some people, lead to the production of more ApoB carrying low-density lipoprotein (LDL) particles and reduce uptake of LDL receptors in the liver. This, in turn, can raise the risk of developing cardiovascular disease. The overconsumption of saturated fat can also contribute to a fatty liver, which, in turn, can lead to a host of problems, mostly notably insulin resistance.

A fat liver does not conjure a particularly beautiful image, but it serves as a nice literary transition as this section is not focused on dietary fat. It addresses body fat.

It's quite tempting to excoriate fat for its inflammatory villainy. Let's first extoll some of its nobler attributes.

1. **Fat is a protective cushion.** A human baby is born with approximately 15 percent body fat, a higher percentage than any other species in the world. Human babies are rather helpless and clumsy creatures. Even when they start crawling and toddling, they are apt to tumble and fall. However, they rarely, if ever, get injured, thanks to their considerable subcutaneous layer of fat.

2. **Fat stores energy.** Adipocytes (fat cells) stockpile energy in the form of triglycerides. Warehoused energy comes in handy for periods of scarcity that were common in our hunter-gatherer days. When the body senses low energy, the pancreas will release the hormone glucagon. Glucagon, will

among other things, trigger a process of lipolysis in which triglycerides are broken down into fatty acids, some of which become ketones, for the body to use as energy.

3. **Fat produces hormones.** Indeed, one of the unsung functions of fat is that it is an endocrine organ. It mostly famously produces the "satiety" hormone named leptin that I will address in the hormones section. Fat also produces the less-heralded adipokines adiponectin and resistin that have their own yang-yin rapport as accelerators and decelerators of metabolic function. Dr. William Li elaborates brilliantly on these hormones in his book *Eat to Beat Your Diet*.
4. **Fat is a furnace.** Fat, specifically brown fat, is responsible for the process of thermogenesis, also known as warming yourself up when you get cold. Your core body temperature hovers in a Goldilocks zone, around 98.6 degrees. When it drops, your brown fat cells go into energy production overdrive to upregulate your core temperature.

White Fat

The majority of adipocytes in your body can be categorized as white fat. White fat checks the boxes on three of the aforementioned four virtues. White fat cells can provide some insulation, but they will not generate heat because they have a low volume of mitochondria. It is the concentration of mitochondria in brown fat that is responsible for its color. The brown hue is due to the prevalence of iron that is needed to synthesize heme and iron-sulfur compounds that are needed for energy production.

White fat generally falls into two categories: subcutaneous fat and visceral fat.

Subcutaneous fat in the body is located under the skin and above the muscle. It's generally the fat you can pinch. It is primarily located in the hips, butt, and thighs. Subcutaneous fat is not as treacherous as visceral fat, but too much is not profitable. More fat requires the production of more blood vessels. Over the long haul, this taxes the heart. Too much subcutaneous fat can also be an indicator that you have too much visceral fat. Visceral fat lies deep within your abdominal cavity and surrounds your organs. It is possible to be thin on the outside and fat on the inside. Dr. Robert Lustig, famous for his video *Sugar: The Bitter Truth*, which unveils the hazards of sugar consumption, dubs this condition "T.O.F.I."[5]

Visceral fat can have very harmful effects on your health. It can lead to insulin resistance, which creates a vicious cycle of generating more and more adipose tissue as glucose is rejected by cells and converted to triglycerides that require more fat storage. The accumulation of fat is a primary culprit in decelerating your metabolism. In fact, a paper published in *Science* in 2021 maintains that metabolic rate remains almost exactly the same from age 20 to 60.[6] This completely debunks the myth that metabolism naturally slows with age. The determinant responsible for slowing metabolism appears to be excess adiposity. Obese individuals are 80 times more likely to develop type 2 diabetes.[7]

Additionally, visceral fat secretes inflammatory cytokines that can accelerate the development of cardiovascular disease and dementia.

The combination of inflammation and insulin resistance can create friendly terrain for cancer development. Inflammation is going to depress immune system functionality, compromising cancer-fighting immune cells' ability to identify and neutralize tumor cells. Insulin resistance will stress the pancreas to produce more of it. High insulin levels can lead to the overproduction of growth factors, which can spark the proliferation of malignant cells.

Brown Fat

Brown fat in newborns is located in their back, neck, and shoulders. During childhood and adolescence, it begins to disperse around the body. By adulthood, brown fat can be found around the neck, kidneys, adrenal glands, heart, and chest. As mentioned, brown fat is rich in mitochondria and serves as the body's furnace, upregulating core temperature through energy production when the body gets cold.

Triggering thermogenesis in your brown fat can actually "beige" your white fat. Cold showers and ice baths, as described, can lead to mitobiogenesis, the creation of new mitochondria, in your white fat. Consuming turmeric, green tea, chili peppers, fish oil, resveratrol, berberine, and cinnamon also may boost activity and induce the "beiging" of white fat.

CHAPTER 12

SWEATING IT OUT

Deliberate Heat Therapy

Give me the power to produce fever, and I will cure all disease.

— Hippocrates

Getting me into a sauna, unlike the ice plunge, requires no arm twisting. The dry heat feels like my natural habitat. I was likely a lizard in a past incarnation, cold-blooded and sun-loving.

A few drops of eucalyptus oil diffused in water and ladled over hot stones produces an aerosol mist that puts me immediately at ease.

While most everyone can avail themselves of a stream of cold water, take a walk, and not eat, access to a sauna can be limited for many people. Unless, of course, you're Finnish. Fortunately for me, my beloved is Finnish (and quite often she feels finished with me). Nevertheless, Schuyler has provided me with a beautiful cedar barrel sauna for which I am deeply grateful. That said, I have also snuggled myself into an affordable infrared sauna blanket, like a hot dog in a bun. They are available for as little as $100.

The legendary Greek physician Hippocrates (c. 460–c. 370 B.C.E.), also known as the "father of medicine," was not alone in recognizing the power of heat to heal. Thermal baths, mud pits, and hot air caverns linked to volcanic sources were all common practices in ancient Egypt dating back to 500 B.C.E. Heated sand and warm baths were used for the treatment of edema, otherwise known as dropsy or fluid retention, in ancient Rome.[1]

Deliberate heat therapies have been utilized around the world for millennia, including saunas in Finland, onsens in Japan, banyas in Russia, hammams in Turkey, and sweat lodges in Native American culture.

While Ffej didn't build structures specifically for the purpose of heat exposure, he endured high daytime temperatures on the savannah. The ability to tolerate a hot climate was crucial in order to accomplish his daily activities. Other hunter-gatherer tribes like the San lived in parts of the Kalahari Desert where they faced extreme temperature fluctuations. Survival in such environments required not only physiological adaptations but also profound knowledge of the environment, including where to find water and how to secure food under harsh conditions.

Most of the current data we have on saunas comes from Finland, which is purported to have more than 2 million of them in a land with 5.5 million people[2]—a novelty statistic only rivaled by New Zealand, which boasts more than five sheep for every citizen.[3] I've become quasi codependent with my cedar barrel sauna, whom I visit every morning. I never tire of her perhaps because the womblike experience that she delivers is erased from memory by the cold stream of 50-degree water that I stand in miserably after every session.

A sauna also provides a very private environment in which to practice otherwise embarrassing rituals. I am apt to chant in the sauna. The sound reverberates nicely. I stretch and breathe and meditate. I often lose myself staring at the grain in the cedar planks and the marvelous organic patterns they make. I move through my own clunky version of hot yoga, descending into a deep knee squat and then popping up into a standing position with a mammoth exhale. I repeat this action until my quads are burning as hot as the stones. At the risk of losing your readership, I must divulge that I am doing all this naked. I promise to never resurface that image.

Frequency matters when it comes to sauna bathing. Four to seven sessions per week confer the maximum benefits, including a 50 percent reduction in all-cause mortality.[4]

The sauna, as we will soon discover, is not just a simply hot room but rather a gateway to unlock myriad adaptive mechanisms in the body. The benefits of regular sauna use are multifarious, as I will now outline.

The Benefits

Cardiovascular Health & Inflammation

Deliberate heat therapy mimics low-grade exercise, raising heart and respiratory rate. While baking like a tuber in the oven of a sauna will not deliver the same level of cardiovascular benefit as a vigorous tennis match, it does provide many of the same perks related to heart health and inflammation levels that I will enumerate with significant loquacity when we talk about exercise in Chapter 13. Here's a very brief preview.

Aerobic exercise improves cardio-metabolic health, making your heart muscle stronger and enhancing your heart's ability to get oxygen to cells for energy production. Your brain specifically benefits from the perfusion of oxygen as it is a gas guzzler when it comes to energy consumption.

Additionally, physical activity as mimicked by sauna use decreases resting heart rate and blood pressure and reduces the development of type 2 diabetes by improving glucose tolerance and insulin sensitivity and decreasing circulating lipid concentrations.

Heat Shock Proteins

Regular deliberate heat therapy activates the production of numerous health-conferring proteins, including heat shock proteins (or HSPs).

These proteins help to maintain the three-dimensional structure of other proteins. Remember there are hundreds of thousands of proteins in the human body, from enzymes to neurotransmitters, from peptide hormones to skeletal muscle. When proteins are produced by the ribosomes in a cell, they undergo a physical process of "folding" in which the protein chain is translated into a three-dimensional structure. The correct three-dimensional structure of proteins is crucial to their function.

Do you remember fashioning paper airplanes during history class? If you didn't pleat the wing aerodynamically, then it wouldn't fly. Similarly, the failure to fold proteins into proper structures generally produces inactive proteins.

What's more is that misfolded proteins can be toxic. For example, let's consider Alzheimer's, the world's most common neurodegenerative disease and form of dementia. Alzheimer's is often characterized by protein misfolding.

Beta-amyloid and tau proteins misfold and aggregate to form amyloid plaques and tangles that are the hallmarks of the disease. These plaques and tangles that strangle neurons and their connections may be more of a symptom of dementia than a cause. Still, protein misfolding is concomitant with aging. Heat shock proteins inhibit the misfolding of proteins and may be helpful in the prevention of Alzheimer's.[5] In this sense, sauna use can keep your noggin from sloggin'.

BDNF

Another sauna-activated molecule is brain-derived neurotrophic factor (commonly known as BDNF), a protein that supports the survival and functionality of existing neurons and stimulates the growth and differentiation of new brain cells and synapses. It serves as a type of fertilizer for the brain, supporting the growth of new neurons and the connections between them.

Low levels of BDNF have been linked to myriad neurological and psychiatric disorders, including depression, schizophrenia, and Alzheimer's disease. Conversely, increasing levels of BDNF through sauna (and exercise) has been shown to improve cognitive function and reduce the symptoms of these ghastly conditions.

Detoxification

When your body is exposed to the high heat of a sauna, your core body temperature can increase as much as 1.8 degrees Fahrenheit.[6] Your internal thermostat turns on and begins the process of thermoregulation. You, along with horses, monkeys, and hippos, can cool down through perspiration.

Heat causes blood vessels to dilate, increasing blood flow to the skin, the largest organ of your body. Sweat, which consists of 99 percent water, emanates out of your skin through millions of miniscule holes called pores. When the sweat hits the air, it turns from a liquid to a vapor. As the sweat evaporates off your skin, you cool down. The human ability to sweat is a secret weapon. The cooling mechanism provides humans with incredible endurance. Even Usain Bolt cannot outrun a cheetah in a 100-yard dash, but across marathon distances, perspiration gives humans a distinctive advantage—one that proved extremely handy when tracking game. In order to dissipate heat, most animals must resort to panting, which is much less efficient than sweating. This gives humans an upper hand in persistent hunting.

A side note: perspiration, on its lonesome, does not render you malodorous. Sweat has no scent at all. You might notice that there is no bouquet to the sweat on your forearm. Body odor is generated when bacteria metabolizes sweat into fragrant fatty acids. And bacteria like to sequester in your armpit and in other ripe crevices.

Sweat carries with it trace amounts of toxic compounds, including phthalates found in fragrances, nail polish, cosmetics, and paints; bisphenol A (BPA) found in clear plastics; and heavy metals, including arsenic, cadmium, lead, and mercury. In this manner, sauna bathing does provide some detoxification. That said, most detoxification responsibilities fall on to the kidneys and the liver.

Stacking Heat & Cold Therapy (Contrast Bathing)

Sauna, especially in combination with deliberate cold-water therapy, can move lymph fluid more readily around the body. The lymph fluid transports toxins to the liver. The practice of contrast bathing in which you alternate between the sauna and cold therapy produces a back and forth of vasodilation and vasoconstriction. This counterposing action increases circulation of the lymph fluid, further aiding in detoxification.

NRF2

Let me celebrate one more impossibly long-named protein. Nuclear factor erythroid 2-related factor 2 (a.k.a. NRF2) is a protein that plays a critical role in regulating the body's antioxidant response. It activates genes that produce antioxidant enzymes such as glutathione and superoxide dismutase (SOD), which help to protect cells from damage caused by free radicals. Free radicals, which are also known as reactive oxygen species, are a natural by-product of energy production. Their production is also a knock-on impact of exposure to X-rays, ozone, cigarette smoking, air pollutants, and caustic industrial chemicals. The high reactivity of free radicals is due to the presence of one unpaired electron that they not-so-generously try to donate to other molecules. Or they may try to pilfer one in order to stabilize.

Free radicals can, at times, serve a beneficial purpose: killing pathogens. However, an overabundance of free radicals like hydrogen peroxide and hydroxyl radical can lead to oxidative stress. Oxidative stress can damage DNA and contribute to a wide range of serious neurodegenerative and psychiatric disorders, including cancer, heart failure, and Parkinson's disease.

Several studies have shown that sauna usage can activate NRF2, leading to an increase in the aforementioned antioxidants. These antioxidants give up some of their own electrons. In making this grand gesture, they act as a natural off switch to the free radical.

Mood Regulation

Deliberate hyperthermia—purposefully making yourself hot—has significant implications on depression and mood regulation. Sauna can activate the production of different compounds that contribute to a sense of euphoria, which may explain my proclivity to immediately get nude. Sauna heightens energy levels and provides relief from pain.

Sauna activates a significant release of the neuropeptide hormone and neurotransmitter dopamine. Dopamine is famously known as the feel-good neurotransmitter. More accurately, it's part of your brain's reward system. It provides motivation to double-down on whatever pleasurable activity in which you may be engaged. The human brain is hardwired to seek out behaviors that release dopamine. Simply, when you're doing something pleasurable, your brain releases a large amount of dopamine. And then you feel good and seek more of that feeling.

This phenomenon is a double-edged sword in modern culture because there are so many maladaptive options that provide neural rewards, including the junkiest of foods, opioids, and other nefarious narcotics. Dopamine foraging on social media can also keep people on the hedonic treadmill of seeking more and more likes and followers. Sauna, on the contrary, is a patently adaptive behavior.

Another category of molecule that is released during sauna bathing is endorphins. Endorphins are peptides, short strings of amino acids, produced in the brain that block the perception of pain and increase feelings of well-being. They are produced and stored in the pituitary gland of the brain. The etymology of the term *endorphin* has its origins in the combination of the words *ENDOgenous*, or occurring naturally in the body, and *morPHINe*, an opium-derived analgesic narcotic. In essence, your body is its own drug lab, cooking up endorphins. The level of endorphins released during sauna bathing can be three times normal, similar to a vigorous jog. In fact, the addictive nature of the runner's high may also apply to regular sauna users. I may be living proof of this hypothesis.

Protocols

In order to harvest the benefits of sauna usage, frequency, duration, and temperature are highly relevant. Here's what the current data supports:[7]

- Frequency: 4–7 sessions per week
- Session duration: 20 minutes
- Temperature: 170–190 degrees Fahrenheit
- Humidity: 10–20 percent

If you do not have access to a sauna, you can purchase a sauna blanket for around $100. The experience is less enjoyable as you are stuffed into the blanket like a hot dog in a bun. But the benefits are likely the same.

Do infrared saunas work as well as traditional saunas? The short answer is . . . probably, but we don't know. There is much more clinical research data available for traditional saunas.

Dry saunas heat the air which, in turn, heats the body. Infrared saunas heat the body directly through infrared radiation. Infrared waves penetrate the body more deeply and can produce benefits at lower temperatures. The benefits might also be slightly different. For example, because it can penetrate the body so deeply, infrared radiation may stimulate the production of melatonin at the subcellular level.

Further, infrared saunas may feel more comfortable for people as temperatures range from 110 to 135 degrees Fahrenheit instead of 175 to 200 degrees Fahrenheit. Personally, I prefer the higher temperatures.

As with all forms of adversity mimetics, you should always consult your physician before adopting a protocol. And ease your way into it.

Specific contraindications for sauna usage include:

- Alcohol consumption (sorry, no beers in the sauna!)
- Whether you are prone to low blood pressure
- Whether you've had a recent heart attack or stroke or are experiencing chest pain
- Young children (who haven't developed good thermoregulation yet)
- If you are pregnant

THE BODY IN BALANCE

Dopamine & . . . Dopamine

Dopamine is the Jekyll and Hyde of neurotransmitters, displaying both excitatory and inhibitory characteristics. It is most notable for its involvement with how we feel pleasure. It also is present in response to patently unpleasurable experiences, such as touching a scorching tea kettle, presumably training the brain to avoid them in the future. In this sense, dopamine plays a major role in neuroplasticity, helping to rewire the brain in response to stimuli.

Dopamine is curiously both yang and yin.

Dopamine can excite and inhibit action potentials depending on the type of dopamine receptor it binds to. In the brain, there are several different types of dopamine receptors, named D1 through D5. The activation of the D1-like family, which includes the D1 and D5 receptors, generally leads to excitatory effects, increasing the likelihood of an action potential. Conversely, the activation of the D2-like family, which includes the D2, D3, and D4 receptors, generally leads to inhibitory effects, decreasing the likelihood of an action potential.

Dopamine is often called the feel-good neurotransmitter because it's associated with feelings of motivation and reward. It is released when we experience something pleasurable (like gorging on truffle fries or making illicit whoopee), which motivates us to seek out these enjoyable experiences again. More fries, please.

The double-edged sword of dopamine lies in that it is not at all discerning between what is adaptive and maladaptive when it comes to pleasure and motivation. For example, dopamine levels can increase in response to the consumption of some healthy foods such as bananas, green leafy vegetables, nuts and seeds, legumes such as lentils and chickpeas, and dark chocolate. Fish, beef, and poultry can also boost dopamine levels because they contain the amino acid tyrosine, which is dopamine's precursor. Health-conferring activities such as exercise and cold-water therapy can also stimulate the adaptive release of dopamine.

At the same time, sugar consumption can also trigger the discharge of dopamine in the brain. This is because scarfing brownies can be quite a satisfying experience, and dopamine is associated with feelings of pleasure and reward. When you eat sugary foods, your taste buds activate and send signals to your brain, as do the neuropods in your gut through the vagus nerve.

In response, your brain releases dopamine, leading to feelings of pleasure. This is part of the reason why cookies and ice cream can be so appealing and why some people may feel a sense of craving or "addiction" to sugary foods. This biological phenomenon is the target of exploitation by Big Food, who nefariously engineer foods to trigger a dopamine response.

Repeated stimulation of the reward system by consuming sugar-laden foods can lead to desensitization. This means that over time, more sugar is needed to activate the dopamine pathways and produce the same pleasurable effect, which can unfortunately contribute to overeating and the development of obesity, and potentially, to the onset of type 2 diabetes.

Certain prescription medications, such as Adderall and Ritalin (used to treat attention-deficit/hyperactivity disorder) and certain antidepressants can increase dopamine levels. Many illicit drugs, like cocaine, methamphetamine, and MDMA, also dramatically increase dopamine quantities.

Both nicotine and alcohol can increase dopamine concentrations, contributing to their addictive properties. This is part of the reason why these substances are so highly addictive. In fact, it's not really more nicotine or cocaine that we seek. It's the dopamine. It operates like a drug of which we are in constant pursuit, and, of course, this can lead to addictive and destructive behavior.

In a way, dopamine is like fire that can be leveraged for both positive purposes like cooking or negative ones like arson. Dopamine in the brain is a reward that trains us to seek out pleasurable experiences—both adaptive and maladaptive. Choosing the right triggers is up to us.

CHAPTER 13

JOINING THE RESISTANCE

Exercise & Strength Training

Not less than two hours a day should be devoted to exercise, and the weather should be little regarded.

— Thomas Jefferson

Mrs. Brody put the fear of God in me. Given my devout atheism, that's a high bar to clear.

Mrs. Brody was the head of physical education at South School in New Canaan, Connecticut, where I matriculated in the third grade.

One dare not call her a gym teacher for the risk of being dispatched to run dozens of punitive laps around the schoolyard.

However, given that she's likely dead now, I can be honest about it. She was a cruel and callous *gym teacher*. There . . . I finally said it.

Mrs. Brody wore the same uniform every day: high-waisted black slacks and a tight-fitting referee jersey that accentuated her enormous, preternaturally high breasts. Affixed to her wrist was a whistle that she never hesitated to fill with air.

Her gray bob, doused in hairspray, remained motionless as she vaulted over pommel horses and swung from the rings. I suppose, in retrospect through a kinder lens, she was impressive for a 60-year-old broad, perhaps even a portrait of '80s feminism. But . . . she was still a mean *gym teacher*.

Anyhow, Mrs. Brody supervised the ghastly annual Presidential Fitness Test. Now disbanded, a good 40 years too late, this national program consisted of a variety of physical tests, including sit-ups, sprints, a mile run, touching your toes, and—the worst—the dreaded pull-up.

Our motley class congregated on the playground one spring afternoon for the test. Each student was distributed a paper leaflet upon which to register his or her performance in each category. Based upon his or her score, each student was then classified in one of four groups—the names of which I have mostly blocked out as I was teetering between the lowest two classifications, standard and substandard. It all came down to the pull-up.

If you qualified for the top tranche, Mrs. Brody would publicly recognize you in the school assembly. This fleeting fame was generally reserved for the broad-shouldered, crew-cutted lacrosse boys and a few bendy gymnasts.

My eyes were not focused anywhere near the top category nor was municipal recognition a reward I sought. My sole concern was simply to avoid being categorized as "substandard." My flaccid ego had suffered enough. I was more than willing to accept "standard" and move the fuck on. In order to do so, however, I needed to perform one solitary pull-up. Unfortunately, the pitiful truth was that I couldn't do it. Well, unless I jumped up from the ground as I attempted to heave my jowls above the bar—which I more or less did.

Given that I had a double-chin, I thought there was a good argument that I had performed two. But to remain credible, I indicated "one" pull-up on my scorecard. This accomplishment was just barely enough to achieve my life goal—to be "standard."

At the end of the test, Mrs. Brody blew her bloody whistle with the zeal of Dizzy Gillespie, collected everyone's leaflets, and gathered the class back in the gymnasium. She paged through the scorecards, perusing them, occasionally raising an eyebrow. And then she paused and fixed her wicked gaze on me.

"Jeff . . . Kras-no," she uttered slowly, enunciating each syllable like Annie Cresta from the Hunger Games.

No fucking way! I thought to myself, much like Katniss.

"You have indicated on your scorecard that you can perform *one* pull-up."

"Yes, Mrs. Brody," I replied faintheartedly.

"Well, let's see it." She pointed to some uneven bars.

This dare elicited a number of snickers from the class. No, unfortunately, not the candy bar.

Timidly, I lumbered over to the daunting apparatus, assumed a crouch, and then hurled myself toward the wooden crossbar. I clutched it as if it were the world's last hot dog, miraculously hoisted my chin to its level, and plunged quickly back to the floor.

This feat of triumphant ineptitude extracted more snorts and whinnies from the barnyard of mocking kids.

I stared at Mrs. Brody, severe and tight-lipped.

"Okay," she barked officiously. "Standard."

Well, Mrs. Brody, wherever you are, you'll be proud to know that I now do 100 pull-ups every day.

The building of muscle, also known as hypertrophy, is perhaps the most obvious and observable example of Good Stress—which is, at times, synonymous with short-term pain for long-term gain. You stress a bicep by repeatedly lifting a heavy object. Eventually, the muscle fibers tear. The body responds by repairing those microtears, and the muscle grows in size provided it has the proper building blocks.

Old Ffej didn't have an Equinox membership or Peloton bicycle. Nor did he consider physical activity a choice. Moving his body in the great outdoors was compulsory as part of the biological imperative to survive. Ffej's quotidian life was a mix of what we might call today aerobic exercise, strength training, and HIIT (high-intensity interval training).

On an average day, Ffej walked 10 miles per day in search of food. The Hadza people of Tanzania, who are among the few remaining hunter-gatherer populations in the world, still walk seven miles per day in pursuit of daily provisions. The same is true for the !Kung people of the Kalahari Desert in southern Africa. For those who are counting on their iWatch, this would equate to approximately 14,000 daily steps.

While Ffej didn't curl 20-pound dumbbells in front of a mirror, he did climb trees, lug firewood, and build structures. He hunted, fished, and foraged. He crafted tools and shelter. And, at night, he might break out in a furious jig. In addition, from time to time, a predator might press Ffej into an involuntary life-preserving sprint that might qualify today as high-intensity interval training.

By mere dint of his lifestyle, Ffej burned between 2,500 and 4,000 calories per day. His quotidian activity in combination with his nutrient-dense and protein-rich diet informed his lithe but sinewy physique.

Chopping wood and carrying water in regular, everyday life conferred many benefits, including superlative cardiovascular health. In fact, in Ffej's era, heart disease was essentially nonexistent, as were diabetes and dementia.

Fast forward to today and heart disease is the world's number one assassin. One of the contributing factors to the development of vascular disease is, of course, physical inactivity and sedentariness. According to the CDC, approximately 75 percent of U.S. adults are not meeting the federal guidelines for both aerobic and muscle-strengthening activity.[1] The key CDC guidelines for adults include at least 150 minutes a week of moderate-intensity exercise or 75 minutes a week of vigorous-intensity aerobic physical activity.[2] In addition, adults should also do muscle-strengthening activities of moderate or greater intensity that involve all major muscle groups on two or more days a week. While these guidelines are not particularly onerous, only one in five Americans manage to hit the mark.

I was always a regular exerciser, even in my more indolent days. However, like many folks, I exercised largely out of guilt. The gym was a form of penance. I was a sinner huffing and puffing his Hail Marys to atone for his overindulgences. I believed that I could set things right by panting on the treadmill for an hour. I now call this misguided approach to exercise "chronic cardio." It's not that aerobic exercise is bad. But, on its own, without other forms of exercise and a focus on eating habits, it will not yield the desired results.

Furthermore, like so many others, I product-ized exercise. It became another bullet on my to-do list. After eight hours of sitting, staring into a screen, I'd haul myself to the gym for an hour. This tendency to cubbyhole exercise as an event instead of integrating movement organically into one's life doesn't work. We've seen a massive efflorescence of gyms in the United States over the last 50 years. But despite there being more than 45,000 dedicated places to sweat and grunt, obesity rates have tripled since the mid-70s.

While I will dive into the particulars of aerobic and resistance training in the pages ahead, the first key to health is changing one's understanding of exercise. We can't treat exercise as an isolated daily event. To live more like Ffej, we must move throughout the day. Modern medicine has given this concept a fancy rubric: N.E.A.T. This acronym stands for non-exercise activity thermogenesis. N.E.A.T. includes all the energy expenditures across the course of your day, from taking the stairs to doing household chores to rucking your groceries. Movement as a way of life has immeasurable benefits—particularly for the old ticker.

The Benefits

Cardio-Metabolic Health

We have all heard countless times that exercise is important for cardio-metabolic health. But why? Most of us have a dull understanding . . . but let's sharpen it.

The human body—more specifically, the mitochondria in your cells—produces energy or ATP that animates everything you do, from reading this book to the unconscious digestion contemporaneously occurring in your gut. The bottom line here: you need to make energy at the level of the cell or you die.

The production of ATP, as we have discussed in prior chapters, is known as cellular respiration. The process has three stages: glycolysis, the Krebs cycle, and the electron transport chain.

Glycolysis is a form of anaerobic metabolism. In other words, this first stage of cellular respiration does not require oxygen to produce energy. Instead, it leverages a process known as fermentation, a process that oenophiles, like myself, are familiar with. Except fermentation in the human body produces lactic acid and not ethyl alcohol as a by-product. It's not totally dissimilar from a sourdough starter whose wild yeast ferments glucose (from flour) and produces carbon dioxide and lactic acid (which contributes to the "sour" taste).

Glycolysis uses glucose to produce a rather trivial amount of ATP. The reason why you start gasping for air when you, for example, scale a steep hill is because your cells are desperate for the oxygen they need to make more energy. When your cells cannot access the requisite oxygen for aerobic respiration, they default to this less efficient process of fermentation. Eventually, you hit a wall and cannot continue because you cannot meet the energy demands of the task.

The second two stages of energy production are aerobic. Hence, they require oxygen. The overwhelming majority of ATP is produced in the final stage. Oxygen serves as the final electron acceptor in the electron transport chain to form H_2O, which, along with CO_2, are the by-products of energy production. I'd be remiss not to point out that these waste products of human cellular respiration are the very requirements of the plant kingdom for the process of photosynthesis. And, of course, the by-product of photosynthesis is oxygen. This symbiosis, also known as the carbon cycle, serves as a reflection of our miraculous coevolution with plants.

When you inhale, millions of air sacs in the lungs fill with freshly oxygenated air. The oxygen then moves into the blood by passing through the very thin walls of the air sacs and then into the capillaries. This process is called diffusion.

It is then the job of the heart to pump blood out through the arteries such that oxygen gets to your cells for energy production. Hemoglobin, an iron-containing transport protein in red blood cells, serves as oxygen's delivery man, supplying oxygen to the cells. When the hemoglobin finishes its delivery, it then becomes a magnet for carbon dioxide, which is a waste product of the cell. Hemoglobin then picks up carbon dioxide and schleps it back to the lungs, where it leaves the body when we exhale.

How efficiently the body accomplishes this transfer is central to cardiovascular health. Aerobic exercise improves this process in myriad ways.

Like curls propel hypertrophy in the biceps, aerobic exercise makes your heart stronger. The heart is a muscle, and like other muscles, it benefits from exercise. A stronger heart can pump more blood with each beat, allowing it to work more efficiently. This leads to a decrease in heart rate both at rest and during physical exertion while also improving blood circulation and lowering blood pressure.

Exercise also stimulates the production of nitric oxide, a molecule that helps blood vessels relax and dilate, thereby improving blood flow and decreasing the stress on arterial walls. And exercise decreases visceral adiposity and lowers plasma triglycerides and serum glucose levels.

Strenuous aerobic exercise improves a key longevity metric known as VO_2 max. VO_2 max measures the maximum rate of oxygen consumption attainable during physical exertion. Superior oxygen consumption reflects cardiorespiratory fitness. A higher VO_2 max means that your body is better at taking oxygen from the air and delivering it to your muscles.

Efficient oxygen delivery is also paramount for cognitive health. Your neurons require energy too. Poor oxygen delivery, also known as ischemia, is highly associated with dementia and Alzheimer's. In many ways, these diseases can be understood as inefficient energy production in the brain.

This brief explanation of the basic mechanisms behind the cardio-metabolic benefits of exercise will surely make you appear intelligent at your next cocktail party.

Exercise & Inflammation

The impact of exercise on inflammation is a portrait of the body's innate homeostatic drive.

Inflammation is a normal immune system reaction to stimuli. Acute bouts of exercise can induce short-term inflammation, elevating levels of pro-inflammatory cytokines like interleuken-6 and TNF-Alpha. Surely, you've seen photos of athletes submerged in postgame ice baths as a means to reduce inflammation.

However, while exercise induces a temporary inflammatory response, over the long haul, moving your body lowers inflammatory levels. In this manner, exercise is exemplary of this book's primary thesis: short-term acute stress results in long-term benefit as the body bounces back. This is good news since chronic inflammation is associated with multiple diseases, including obesity and cardiovascular disease.

One of the reasons for exercise's beneficial impact on inflammation centers around its ability to oxidize fat and neutralize its inflammatory tendencies. Excess visceral fat, often due to overnutrition and insulin resistance, is inflammatory and atherogenic. Adipocytes (fat cells) release inflammatory molecules, leading to meta-inflammation, a chronic agitation of the immune system. Excess immune activation caused by obesity is of particular concern for vascular health as it drives the production of foam cells in the arteries and the progression of atherosclerosis.

A little more on inflammation and vascular disease by analogy with hockey. You want your arteries and veins to function like an ice rink just after the Zamboni has passed over. You drop a puck on a freshly resurfaced rink and it glides effortlessly on the ice. After a brutal hockey game, the rink has been all marked and pitted up by the skates of ruffians, often Canadian in descent. You drop a puck on pockmarked ice and it barely budges. Similarly, when your vascular system is smooth, blood flows easily and oxygen gets delivered to your cells without much fuss. But when arteries are scarred by inflammation, particles, specifically cholesterol-toting ApoB molecules, are more likely to get stuck in the endothelium, the layer between the bloodstream and the arteries, and form plaques and potential blockages.

This unfortunate circumstance prohibits blood from efficiently carrying oxygen to cells and impedes energy production. An inadequate blood supply to an organ or part of the body is called ischemia.

The deposition of plaques in arterial walls is called atherosclerosis. Atherosclerosis comes from the Greek words *athero* meaning "gruel" or "paste" and *sclerosis*, meaning "hardness." A gruel-like hardness in your vascular system instinctively sounds like a condition to avoid. Indeed, when atherosclerosis narrows the arteries close to your heart, you may develop coronary artery disease, which can cause chest pain (angina), a heart attack (myocardial infarction), or heart failure.

Bottom line: you want to minimize vascular inflammation. Exercise contributes to that project, earning yet another feather in its formidable cap.

The Brain & Mood Regulation

Exercise is most famously associated with the release of endorphins, naturally occurring opioids, which promote both a feeling of well-being and the minimization of pain. (I delved more deeply into the cheery world of endorphins in Chapter 11 on deliberate heat therapy.)

Interestingly, there is new emerging data about a series of small proteins called myokines. Myokines are produced and released by skeletal muscle cells in response to muscular contraction. This phenomenon points to the new understanding of muscle as a secretory organ. There are myokine receptors on many organs including the liver, pancreas, heart, and brain.

BDNF, also covered in the heat therapy chapter, is a myokine and both maintains the function of neurons and contributes to neuro biogenesis (the production of new brain cells). We know that aerobic exercise in humans is associated with significant structural alterations in the brain, promoting neurogenesis and improving synaptic transmission in the hippocampus. Further, regular exercise is associated with better consistent sleep quality, which improves mood and memory. These mechanisms may all be mediated by the newly discovered muscle "secretome."

Mitochondrial Biogenesis

Exercise induces adaptations in several cell types throughout the body. Moving your body activates mitochondrial biogenesis (the production of new mitochondria) in fat cells as well as in skeletal muscle and heart cells, thus increasing aerobic respiration (energy production) within these tissues. Like deliberate cold therapy, exercise can also beige your white fat. Remember, earth tones are the preferred tint of fat.

At a very basic level, all you do is make energy—until you don't. Given that energy is generated in your mitochondria, you want to do everything you can to ensure their functionality and produce new ones. Mitobiogenesis is purportedly due to activation of AMPK, the pathway that I described in the fasting section. Novel mitochondria stimulate energy generating processes, increasing glucose uptake and fatty acid oxidation. These exercise-induced enhancements of mitochondrial function are important in preventing cardiovascular dysfunction. You want energy production in your heart cells to be optimal.

A healthy heart readily utilizes fatty acids. An ailing heart is associated with a shift toward glucose metabolism in order to preserve cardiovascular function. However, over time, this shift may ultimately result in myocardial insulin resistance, impairing glucose uptake and accelerating cardiovascular dysfunction.

Resistance Training & Sarcopenia

There are few adversity mimetics more observable than strength training. We stress biceps muscles, for example, through repeatedly lifting something obscenely heavy. As we near the end of our set, we quite literally microtear the muscle's fibers, and, in response, the body repairs the microtears by adding amino acids, namely actin and myosin, to the myofilament of the muscle, which causes it to grow in size. Through the progressive overload of the muscle, you get stronger and soon find yourself doing your best Marky Mark impersonation in front of the bathroom mirror.

Building muscle is useful beyond mere vanity—especially as we age. The gradual loss of muscle mass, strength, and function is known as sarcopenia. On average, we lose 1 percent of our muscle mass per year starting in middle age.[3] Over time, this adds up.

We've all seen elderly folk struggle to haul themselves out of chairs. The failure of muscle function reduces the ability to perform daily tasks and live autonomously. It is also a major factor in falls and fractures, as well as hospitalizations and surgeries, which increase the risk of complications.

In fact, the in-hospital mortality rate is 28.6 percent in patients with sarcopenia and 11.0 percent in patients without sarcopenia.[4] Despite the short-term stress and occasional dreariness of weight and resistance training, the long-term benefits are impossible to deny. Maintaining the ability to get up on your own to take a pee should trump whatever aversion you have for the weight room.

Muscle & Blood Glucose Management

It is quite normal to have postprandial (after meal) blood glucose elevation. Carbohydrates are absorbed into the bloodstream through the small intestine, and it takes a moment for the Uber driver to arrive. The cabbie is insulin, of course, and he will take carbo-passengers to one of 30 million destinations. As his GPS searches for its route, glucose is in the bloodstream. One of the best ways to help glucose efficiently find its cellular destination is through exercise.

Muscle use serves as a highly efficient serum glucose vacuum. And, it makes all the sense in the world. If you hit the deck for 30 push-ups after lunch, your muscles will require energy for the task at hand and suck up available sugar from the bloodstream. Even taking a leisurely 10-minute walk after a meal is an effective way to temper any potential glucose spikes.

Further, when a muscle contracts, it does not require insulin to uptake glucose. I witnessed incredible results in my blood glucose levels after approximately three months of resistance training. Like a kid in a candy store, increased muscle mass greedily vacuumed up excess sugar. In combination with fasting and other dietary modifications and well-timed cold therapy, resistance training was the key to reversing my insulin resistance.

Aerobic Training Basics

Each body is different and will respond differently to exercise. Hence, there is no singular regimen that is applicable to everyone. That said, the prevailing wisdom for exercise includes seven sessions per week. This does not necessarily mean that you must exercise every day, but it does point to seven discrete bouts of exercise combining aerobic, resistance, and flexibility training. Let's begin with aerobic training.

In recent years, there has been a lot of attention paid to HIIT, high-intensity interval training, where bursts of near-maximum effort alternate with bouts of lower-intensity exercise. Here's a typical portrait of a HIIT workout:

You begin with a warm-up, spending 5 to 10 minutes doing light aerobic activity to get your muscles warmed up and ready to work. This might include light jogging, cycling at a low intensity, or doing jumping jacks.

The warm-up period is followed by high-intensity exercise. This could be sprinting, cycling at a high intensity, or doing bodyweight exercises like squats or burpees—the routine named after Royal H. Burpee, who created the exercise as part of his Ph.D. thesis in applied physiology from Columbia University in 1940. The intensity of this exercise should be such that you're working near your maximum effort. This could last anywhere from 30 seconds to a couple of minutes.

After the high-intensity exercise, there is a recovery period where you're still moving but at a much lower intensity to catch your breath and prepare for the next high-intensity interval. This could be walking or cycling at a very low intensity. The recovery period is approximately as long as the high-intensity exercise, or potentially longer, again depending on your fitness level.

You repeat this pattern, alternating between high-intensity exercise and recovery periods for the duration of your workout. The number of cycles will depend on your fitness level and the length of your intervals but could range from four to eight repetitions for a beginner and potentially more for an advanced athlete.

After you've completed all your intervals, there is a 5- to 10-minute cooldown period. This could be similar to your warm-up, with light aerobic activity. Stretching can also be beneficial during this period.

A typical HIIT workout is time-efficient with a duration of 10 to 30 minutes, not including warm-up and cooldown. However, because of the high intensity, it can often be very challenging and effective at improving cardiovascular fitness, muscular strength, endurance, and overall metabolic health.

Some sports, like soccer and competitive tennis, mimic HIIT in that they alternate between extreme exertion and low-intensity recovery periods.

While HIIT certainly has benefits, in the past decade, scientists and physiologists have re-embraced the fitness benefits of slow and steady "zone 2" cardio. Zone 2 exercise refers to a specific level of intensity that keeps your heart pumping in the range between 60 and 70 percent of your overall maximum heart rate. In zone 2, you are typically able to have a chat with your mum or a colleague without being out of breath. Though talking with your mum may be enough to raise your heart rate on its own. Everyone's mum is different.

Studies have demonstrated that endurance athletes have greater gains in VO_2 max when incorporating zone 2 than when they only do HIIT and sprint training. Further, it appears that zone 2 exercise is more effective at burning fat than more rigorous activity.

Exercise intensity is characterized by five distinct heart rate zones. As you increase pace and resistance, heart rate increases. At different heart rate zones, your body leverages different fuel sources to create energy for your cells. At lower heart rates (zones 1 and 2), your body primarily uses fat as a fuel source for your muscles. Burning fat is more energetically efficient than burning glucose. And given that we generally have significant stockpiles of fat, we can perform zone 2 exercise for extended periods.

When your heart rate elevates into zones 3 to 5, your body starts to use more glycogen, stored glucose, from your muscles to supplement the fat. As oxygen demand outweighs supply, the body relies on glycolysis—anaerobic respiration—for energy production. This process produces excess lactate, which is associated with muscle fatigue, but, contrary to popular myth, is not related to muscle soreness the next morning.

Hiking, brisk walking, jogging, cycling, and swimming at moderate intensity for at least 30 minutes all qualify as zone 2 cardio.

Aerobic training follows an 80-20 rule: 80 percent of your aerobic training should fall into zone 2 and 20 percent should be at higher intensities. This 80-20 distribution of zone 2 and HIIT makes intuitive sense if you think about the way Ffej and our hunter-gatherer ancestors got exercise. Of course, they weren't huffing and puffing on a treadmill under the watchful eye of a trainer. They maintained their fitness by dint of their normal lifestyle. And 80 percent or more of Ffej's "movement" practice was zone 2 in the form of walking or gathering wood and water. In rare, likely undesirable circumstances, Ffej would be forced into a full sprint. So, if you are considering five sessions of aerobic training per week, earmark four of them for zone 2.

Resistance Training Basics

Resistance training is a method of improving muscular strength and endurance. During resistance training, you work against a force to build muscle and promote bone health. This force can come from your body weight, gravity, bands, weighted bars, dumbbells, or machines.

The goal of resistance training is typically to build muscle for reasons I will enumerate. The body has north of 600 muscles. It would be life-consuming to attempt to train each one. Still, a good resistance training program will be spread across all the major muscle groups, including chest, back, shoulders, arms, abdominals, legs, and hips.

Muscle is built through progressive overload. Progressive overload involves continuously increasing the demands on the musculoskeletal system to continually make gains in muscle size, strength, and endurance. In order to get stronger and build muscle, you need to continuously challenge your body to exceed its preexisting limits.

This principle can be applied in various ways, including increasing the weight you are lifting, increasing the number of sets or repetitions of a certain exercise, increasing the frequency that you train a muscle group, increasing the intensity by taking less respite between sets, and improving your form by performing an exercise with a fuller range of motion.

Progressive overload doesn't mean you should increase the weight, volume, or frequency every time you train. Doing so could lead to overtraining and an increased risk of injury. Instead, it's a gradual process that involves small, incremental increases over time. The main goal is to continually challenge the muscles over time so they get stronger and more efficient.

There are undeniably some aesthetics involved in building muscle. Modern culture celebrates six-pack abdominals, bulging biceps, and chiseled pecs. However, muscle development has benefits far beyond what meets the eye. Obviously, increased muscle mass leads to greater strength, which renders everyday tasks easier and enhances performance in sports and physical activities. It also helps improve mobility and balance, which is particularly important as we age.

Muscle tissue burns more calories at rest than fat tissue does, so having more muscle can help increase your basal metabolic rate, the number of calories your body burns at rest. This can be beneficial for weight management. Muscle also serves as a glucose sink and improves insulin sensitivity. Unlike other cells, muscle cells, when contracted, do not require insulin to uptake glucose. In this way, muscle mass helps to balance blood sugar and insulin levels.

Resistance training also stimulates bone growth, increases bone density, and reduces the risk of osteoporosis. This is crucial, especially for women who are at a higher risk of developing osteoporosis. Strong muscles help maintain better posture and keep the body in alignment, which can prevent various aches and pains, especially in the lower back.

There is also emerging research that demonstrates that muscle cells are involved in mood regulation. When muscles contract, they secrete chemicals into the bloodstream. Among these chemicals are the myokines I mentioned earlier in this chapter, which have been referred to as "hope molecules." These small proteins travel to the brain, cross the blood-brain barrier, and act as an antidepressant.

This book is not the appropriate venue to discuss the nuances of split, goblet, and box squats or prescribe a bench press routine. Those specifics are best left to a certified physiotherapist. A basic resistance training regimen consists of two or three sessions per week and includes an exercise for each major muscle group.

There are two other key components for effective hypertrophy. One is proper nutrition, specifically the consumption of high-quality protein. There are 21 different amino acids in the body. The combination of those amino acids creates certain proteins, including the ones that help build muscle. Of the 21 amino acids, 12 are produced endogenously in the body. Nine are essential. In other words, you need to consume them exogenously. That is, eat them in your diet.

The three essential amino acids most responsible for muscle protein synthesis are known as branched-chain amino acids, or BCAAs. This group is leucine, isoleucine, and valine.

While these amino acids are more bioavailable in meat, you can fulfill all your amino acid requirements in the plant kingdom. You simply need to be more aware of what you are eating.

The other compulsory element of building muscle is adequate recovery time. Muscles actually grow when you're resting, not when you're working out. It's during rest that your body rebuilds and strengthens your muscles. It's essential to get enough sleep and to take rest days between intense workout sessions.

My basic resistance training regimen is 100 pull-ups, 100 push-ups, 100 sit-ups, and 100 simple squats per session. I can do this almost anywhere, whether there's a gym or not. The pull-ups sometimes require a little creativity and often cause my children embarrassment as I am often seeking out scaffolding on family trips for use as a pull-up bar.

Flexibility Basics

Being flexible, broadly in life, is indicative of one's ability to alter plans and adapt to new situations easily. Flexibility allows us to bend to emerging circumstances or requirements. In my chaotic den of daughters, flexibility is a requirement for retaining sanity. You might empathize.

Physiological flexibility can refer to myriad concepts depending on the context. Metabolic flexibility, for example, reflects your body's ability to switch between using carbohydrates or fats as its primary source of energy depending on availability. Neuroplasticity, the brain's ability to reorganize itself by forming new neural connections, demonstrates a form of brain flexibility. Homeostatic flexibility signifies the body's ability to maintain internal balance in response to changes in the external environment.

Physical flexibility most often refers to your body's capacity to move through a range of motion. There are three primary types of flexibility.

- Dynamic flexibility is the ability to perform kinetic movements of the muscles, ligaments, and tendons to bring a limb through its full range of motion.
- Active flexibility is the ability to assume and maintain extended positions using only the tension of the muscle. For example, lifting the leg and keeping it high without any external support other than the leg muscles.
- Passive flexibility is the ability to assume extended positions using only your weight, the support of your limbs, or some other apparatus such as a chair or a barre. The ability to maintain the position does not come solely from your muscles, as it does with active flexibility. Being able to perform the splits is an example of passive flexibility as you are leveraging your body weight against the floor below you.

Increased flexibility can enhance your ability to move freely and easily, making daily activities and physical tasks, from tying your shoelaces to replacing a light bulb, less strenuous. In sport, superior flexibility can enhance performance through greater agility. As an avid tennis player, I always marvel at Novak Djokovic's ability to slide into a full split on a hardcourt to swat back a potential winner.

A flexible muscle is also less likely to become injured if you have to make a sudden move. And, by increasing the range of motion in a particular joint, you can decrease the resistance on your muscles during various activities.

Regular flexibility training can help keep your muscles from becoming tight and short, thus helping to maintain proper alignment, which can lead to better posture. Adequate flexibility can also reduce muscle soreness post-workout.

Stretching is the most common way to increase flexibility. There are two primary types: dynamic stretching and static stretching, each with its own purpose and benefits.

- **Dynamic stretching** involves movement. It is designed to warm up the muscles and increase their range of motion. During dynamic stretching, you gradually increase the speed, intensity, and range of motion of these movements, while always remaining within your normal range. This type of stretching is usually performed prior to a workout to prepare the muscles for physical activity. Examples can include leg swings, arm circles, walking lunges, or torso twists.

- **Static stretching** is performed by stretching a muscle or group of muscles to its farthest point and then maintaining or holding that position for 15 to 60 seconds. Static stretching is typically done after a workout to help cool down the body and improve flexibility. Examples include the hamstring stretch, calf stretch, or triceps stretch.

Post-workout stretching helps in reducing muscle tension and promoting circulation, which aids in the recovery and repair process. Stretching increases blood flow to the muscles. This improved blood circulation can help speed up recovery from muscle and joint injuries.

Yoga is excellent for improving flexibility as it incorporates a variety of poses that stretch and strengthen different parts of the body while also helping calm the mind and reduce stress. Like yoga, Pilates also promotes flexibility while strengthening the muscles.

Here Are Seven Keys to Effective Stretching:

- Consistency: Aim to stretch every day. Regularity is key when it comes to increasing flexibility. Even 10 minutes a day can lead to improvements over time.
- Warm up: Always warm up your body with a few minutes of light cardio activity before you start stretching. This increases blood flow to the muscles and can make them more pliable.
- Go slow and steady: When you stretch, go slow and be gentle. Never force a stretch and avoid bouncing, as it can cause injury. You should feel a stretch, but it shouldn't cause pain.
- Hold stretches: For static stretches, hold each stretch for at least 20 to 30 seconds. It takes time to lengthen tissues safely, and holding a stretch allows the muscles to gradually relax and extend.
- Breathe: Breathing deeply and relaxing during a stretch can help you reach a little deeper into each stretch.
- A full-body approach: Aim for a full-body stretch routine, even if you have specific areas of focus. This can help maintain overall balance in the body.
- Hydration: Staying hydrated can help keep your muscles and connective tissue flexible. Water makes up a whopping 80 percent of the cartilage found in your joints.[5] Without it, its ability to absorb impact can decrease over time. This leads to pain and lack of mobility. If you're exercising vigorously, it is recommended that you drink 80 percent of your body weight in fluid ounces. I weigh approximately 156 pounds, so I would drink approximately 125 ounces, or about a gallon, of electrolyte-infused water daily.

THE BODY IN BALANCE

Energy Balance & Weight Management

Weight management is actually an "exercise" in energy equilibrium. Maintaining a healthy weight involves balancing energy consumed, energy expended, and energy stored.

We stockpile energy as fat. In the section on fasting, I described how storing fat is adaptive—just not ALL the time. Humans were engineered to become a little fat in the late summer and autumn as a bulwark against winter's fallow. It's easy to vilify fat in today's social media culture—but fat is nothing more than warehoused energy.

We simply want to adaptively manage the size of our fat repository. And one way to do this is through exercise.

Exercise is a fundamental component of weight management through various physiological mechanisms. One of the most direct ways exercise helps with weight management is by burning calories. The more intense and prolonged the activity, the more calories are burned.

There's been much debate in recent years around the "calories in and calories out" approach to weight management. Let's poke at it.

First off, what is a calorie?

A calorie is a relatively bizarre and arcane measurement for a unit of energy. In the context of nutrition and exercise, when people refer to calories, they're actually referring to kilocalories (kcal). A kilocalorie is the amount of heat required to raise the temperature of one kilogram of water by one degree Celsius.

Humans get calories from consuming macronutrients in their diet. Carbohydrates provide 4 calories per gram, protein provides 4 calories per gram, and fat provides 9 calories per gram. And I'll add, somewhat wistfully, alcohol, which provides 7 "empty" calories.

So, what is the association between calories and weight management? In order to unpack this, we need to review the basic laws of thermodynamics.

The first law of thermodynamics, also known as the law of conservation of energy, states that energy cannot be created or destroyed, only transferred or converted from one form to another. In terms of calories and human metabolism, this law underlies the concept of energy balance. The calories we consume from food provide us with energy. This energy is either used by the body for activities and bodily functions or stored in the body, mostly as fat. If you consume more calories than your body uses, you will gain weight. If you consume fewer calories than your body uses, you will lose weight.

The second law of thermodynamics states that in any energy transfer or transformation, some amount of energy is lost as heat. In biological systems, this means that not all energy (calories) consumed can be perfectly converted into work or stored energy. Some of the energy is lost as heat during metabolic processes. This is the reason why the body has a basal metabolic rate, which is the minimum amount of energy required to keep the body functioning at rest. This energy is largely used for maintaining body temperature.

In other words, you burn about one calorie per minute lounging on the couch watching *Curb Your Enthusiasm* or sitting at your desk typing gossipy e-mails because your body is maintaining body temperature, digestion, and other basic processes. That totals 1,440 calories burned per day . . . just staying alive.

Alternately, you burn about 100 calories walking a mile at a leisurely pace (about 3 miles per hour). Given Ffej walked on average 10 miles per day, he burned 1,000 calories by mere dint of his daily perambulation.

Generally, the recommended daily calorie intake is 2,000 calories a day for women and 2,500 for men. But, of course, this totally depends on other variables, including physical activity. Despite these recommendations, according to the United Nations Food and Agriculture Organization's latest annual statistics report, the ever-expanding denizens of Europe and North America consumed on average 3,540 calories per day.[6]

Given this, you can very easily see how the elixir of modern sedentariness and overconsumption quickly leads to obesity. The general rule is that 3,500 excess calories will lead to the gain of one pound of fat. So, if your consumption outpaces your burn by 500 calories per day, you will gain a pound of fat every week.

While the laws of thermodynamics absolutely apply to weight management, not all calories are created equal; 100 calories of jelly beans have a very different impact on the body than 100 calories of black beans.

Different foods send different signals to the body. Foods with high levels of fructose, for example, will signal cells to become insulin resistant and store fat.

Calories in fiber are not absorbed into the bloodstream but instead are metabolized by your gut bacteria. So, "you" might only get 90 of the 100 calories in a handful of walnuts. Your gut bugs are the recipients of the balance.

Calories from ketones are actually wasted as you exhale or urinate.

Lastly, macronutrients differ in the amount of energy that is required for their digestion. This is known as the thermic effect of food. Protein is the most thermic macronutrient with approximately 25 to 30 percent of its calories being used for its own digestion.[7]

There are other ways that exercise impacts weight. For example, strength training increases muscle mass. Muscle tissue burns more calories at rest compared to fat tissue. Thus, having a higher muscle-to-fat ratio can boost the body's basal metabolic rate, leading to more calories being burned throughout the day, even when checking Instagram.

Exercise also regulates appetite, relieves stress, and improves sleep—all of which can impact metabolic health and weight management. I could extol the virtues of exercise till doomsday, but I think you get the idea.

CHAPTER 14

FIAT LUX

Light Therapy

O sleep, O gentle sleep, Nature's soft nurse, how have I frightened thee.
That thou no more will weigh my eyelids down,
And steep my senses in forgetfulness?

— WILLIAM SHAKESPEARE, *HENRY IV, PART 2*

Let me begin with an admission. I love to watch movies, documentaries, and a good TV series. It's a guilty pleasure.

Schuyler and I were members of Netflix when they used to send you red DVD-containing envelopes via snail mail. It seems like eons ago that two flirtatious hours of Kate Hudson and Matthew McConaughey would be delivered right to our mail slot. It's difficult to grok the scale of evolutionary history when I can barely remember the era of mail-order romcoms. At that point, I never dreamed of the day when you could cue up *How to Lose a Guy in 10 Days* or *Fool's Gold* on a whim. Of course, now there are hundreds of platforms that offer every conceivable movie, documentary, sporting event, and TV series on an on-demand, 24-7 basis.

And it's just too tempting. You're tired. It's been a long day. You're full from dinner. Just one episode of *Curb Your Enthusiasm* before bed. Or maybe two. After all, it's pretty. . . pretty . . . pretty good.

Watching Larry David hysterically step in his own shit seems innocuous enough. But upon greater inspection, it's not just his awkward hilarity that might be impeding your sleep.

Let's go back 12,000 years and examine the conditions in which our bodies were engineered.

The sunrise generally served as Ffej's alarm clock. This was somewhat dependent on season, but it was not uncommon for Ffej to rouse at the first crack of light. Of course, Ffej did not have blackout curtains on his hut and often slept outside so his exposure to morning light was customary. This habitual contact with early morning sunlight informed certain adaptations.

I'll get deeper into the mechanism of how light impacts physiology in a bit, but here's a primer.

Light exists across a wave spectrum. Humans can see visible light across a sliver of that spectrum between ultraviolet and infrared or between approximately 400 and 700 nanometers. In the morning, when the sun is low, there is a greater prevalence of a slice of the visible light spectrum (closer to ultraviolet) known as blue light. Blue light exists between 380 and 500 nanometers.

When humans take in morning light, blue-light radiation enters the eye and interacts with specialized neurons in the inferior part of the retina. These cells then send a message to your body's timekeeper—two wee nodes just above the roof of your mouth known as the suprachiasmatic nucleus. These nuclei are responsible for setting your circadian clock. *Circa* means "approximately" and *dia* means "day." *Circadian* means "approximately a day."

The suprachiasmatic nucleus regulates the flow of hormones in your body across approximately a day. Specifically, it signals the pineal gland to produce and secrete the hormone melatonin at a certain time.

The morning time is generally characterized by a rise in melatonin's hormonal foil, cortisol, which contributes to the feeling of alertness that you require as you begin your day. I will describe the seesaw relationships between cortisol and melatonin in the "Body in Balance" section.

As the sun set and darkness pervaded, Ffej and his fellow villagers would congregate and commune around a roaring fire. The flames of the fire emit amber light waves closer to infrared. And because the firepit is at ground level, light is being received in the superior part of the retina. The morning light triggers an endocrine response that sets our circadian rhythm, but the evening light has no impact. This is not by mistake. This mechanism evolved as an advantage to maximize alertness during the day and induce sleep at night.

But, yet again, this adaptive mechanism has been upended by the tantalizing lure of Netflix. The glow discharged from your flatscreen, laptop, or iPad is blue light. Viewing blue light at night is upsetting your hormonal balance as the confused suprachiasmatic nucleus doesn't know morning from night except by dint of the signals it receives from the neurons in your retina.

The result is, as the Beastie Boys rapped, "No Sleep Till Brooklyn" or until anywhere else. One in every three Americans report symptoms of insomnia; 10 percent have a chronic insomnia disorder which occurs at least three times per week for at least three months.[1]

Of course, Larry David cannot be blamed for the global scourge of insomnia. Stress, sleep apnea, alcohol, and caffeine overconsumption can also contribute to poor and disrupted sleep.

What are the knock-on impacts of poor sleep? The answer requires an entire article or five—but here's a brief glimpse.

The cumulative long-term effects of sleep loss and sleep disorders have been associated with a wide range of deleterious health consequences, including an increased risk of hypertension, diabetes, obesity, depression, and cardiovascular disease.[2] We also know that memory consolidation appears to take place during REM sleep but don't completely understand why or we can't remember the reason ;-). Sleep also activates the glymphatic system, the brain's version of the lymphatic system, that is responsible for repair of brain tissues. This "glymph" is responsible for cleaning out beta-amyloid proteins that are highly associated with Alzheimer's disease.[3]

Many mysteries regarding sleep remain. At first glance, it appears maladaptive. We're not procreating or eating, and, in slumber, we are susceptible to predation. That said, when we disrupt our circadian balance and homeostatic drive, disease knocks at the door. All the conditions elicited by disrupted sleep, from disease to mere crankiness, should . . . curb your enthusiasm.

Let's take a deeper look into the nature of light.

The sun will come up tomorrow. Little Orphan Annie among others offered us this optimistic reminder. Indeed, light is one of the few things we can count on. It gives dependably and unconditionally. It requires no ether to carry it. It has a singular gear that propels it constantly at 186,300 miles per second.

Photons are units of light that hurtle toward Earth as a product of the fusion of hydrogen nuclei. The one-way travel time of a quanta from sun to Earth is approximately eight minutes. If you were vacationing on Jupiter (nothing I'd recommend, given an average surface temperature of negative 166 degrees Fahrenheit), you'd need to wait an additional 35 minutes to observe the same light packet. And, in that, you've just grokked the theory of relativity (or part of it).

Light is measured in "lux" (Latin for *light*). It's a relatively quaint and antiquated metric. One lux is equivalent to the illumination that would exist on a surface all points of which are one meter from the flame of one candle.

A fully overcast sky at sunrise has about 40 lux. The brightest midday sunlight has over 100,000 lux. The ambient illumination of the sky at sunrise on a clear day hovers around 400 lux.[4]

Humans evolved with sunlight. Our physiology responds to light in myriad ways depending on the kind of light. Light exists across a wavelength spectrum measured in nanometers (or one billionth of a meter). On one side of the spectrum, there is ultraviolet radiation, commonly referred to as UVC, UVB, and UVA, spanning the distance between 100 and 400 nanometers. On the other wing of the spectrum, we have infrared radiation.

Infrared light has wavelengths longer than ultraviolet and visible light but shorter than those of terahertz radiation microwaves. More specifically, infrared light encompasses the following wavelength ranges:

Near-infrared ranges from about 760 nanometers (nm) to about 1400 nm. Short-wavelength infrared ranges from 1400 nm to 3,000 nm. Mid-wavelength infrared ranges from 3,000 nm to 8,000 nm. Long-wavelength infrared ranges from 8,000 nm to 15,000 nm. And far-infrared ranges from 15,000 nm to 1,000,000 nm (or 1 mm).

Stuck in the middle, like the ham in a sandwich, is visible light, the segment of the electromagnetic spectrum that the human eye can see. A typical human eye will respond to wavelengths from about 380 to about 700 nanometers.

Each of these light bands has different properties and different human applications.

Blue Light & Circadian Rhythm

Blue light is a segment of the visible light spectrum between 380 and 500 nanometers.

The amount of blue light in the sky varies throughout the day. However, due to the way our atmosphere scatters sunlight, blue light is particularly noticeable during the "blue hours" of dawn and dusk. The blue hour refers to the period of twilight in the morning and in the evening when the sun is just below the horizon. At these times, indirect sunlight is evenly diffused and can give the sky a blue shade.

Blue light, as I have described, has a specific impact on human circadian rhythm. Our circadian rhythm is famously associated with the sleep-wake cycle but also bears additional responsibilities. It regulates hormone production and secretion, hunger and satiety, metabolism, antioxidant production, and body temperature.

Blue light, specifically in the range between 460 nm and 484 nm, can set your circadian clock. When humans get morning light, blue-light radiation enters the eye and interacts with specialized neurons in the inferior part of the retina known as intrinsically photosensitive retinal ganglion cells. These sensory neurons evolved in the lower part of the retina because light from the sun is coming from above, the superior field.

These cells then send a message to your body's master clock—a pair of small nuclei in the hypothalamus of the brain, above the optic chiasma, known as the suprachiasmatic nucleus. The suprachiasmatic nucleus regulates the flow of hormones in your body across approximately a day. Specifically, it signals the pineal gland to produce and secrete the hormone melatonin at a certain time. Melatonin naturally induces grogginess.

When your eyes get blue light in the morning, your circadian clock is set such that about 12–14 hours later, melatonin will begin to pulse through your bloodstream and round your day with a sleep.

What to Do in the Morning:

The protocol is simple. Within an hour of waking up, get 20 minutes of morning light outdoors. Ideally, you're up before 9 A.M., though this may be difficult for some shift workers. Do not wear sunglasses. You can just survey the scene, look into the lower sky, and, of course, avoid staring directly at the bright ball of gas.

Blue light does not travel effectively through windows. So, steep your tea, put on a jumper, and get outside. A bright day with more lux might require a smaller time commitment. An overcast day will require more patience.

If natural light is not an option due to schedule or geographic location, light-therapy lamps can be used. The lamps are often dubbed SAD lamps as they also address seasonal affective disorder that is common in the winter in the farther reaches of the northern or southern hemispheres.

These lamps provide a measured amount of balanced spectrum light, often around 10,000 lux, and can be used to stimulate a morning light response. Spending 20 minutes approximately 12 inches away from a SAD light box will mimic the effect of the sun.

What (Not) to Do in the Evening:

- Stop looking at screens at least an hour before bedtime. Your intrinsically photosensitive retinal ganglion cells (ipRGCs) are MORE sensitive to blue light at night than in the morning.
- Turn on blue-light filters. Most computers and tablets now have a nighttime filter. Apple's Night Shift uses geolocation and sunset time data to reduce the amount of blue light your device emits.

- If you can withstand the mockery of your children, you can don blue blocker sunglasses that mitigate blue light.
- If you must binge *Succession*, then try to have your eye level above the screen such that you're looking down your nose at Logan Roy. You may already do this for moral reasons. Your blue-light sensitive neurons evolved in the inferior part of your retina. So, while it doesn't eliminate the impact, it's better if the screen is in the inferior field.
- Have amber night lights at floor level for midevening pees. Avoid turning on a harsh overhead light when nature calls.
- While LED lights are more energy efficient than incandescent bulbs, they also produce more blue light. Many companies now produce "amber" LED bulbs, which mitigate some blue light. In general, avoid overhead lighting at night and go dim and amber.
- Blackout curtains or curtains that block overhead light are a solid option for your bedroom.

While we're at it, some other tips for good sleep architecture:

- Try to take your last bite of food three hours before you go to bed. Ideally, you're going to sleep with your food digested. This helps the body maximize its restoration and repair processes.
- Keep it cool: Turn off the heat if you can or set your thermostat between 60 and 66 degrees Fahrenheit.
- Get regular exercise. Nothing too vigorous close to bedtime, though a walk after dinner is key as a glucose sink.

- Meditation. Quiet the mind as you move from the bright, busy yang state of the day into the dark, tranquil yin state of the night. You can use the breath as described in the breathwork section to move into your parasympathetic nervous system. A 4-7-8 pattern, in which you inhale for four counts, hold for seven, and exhale for eight will decrease heart and respiratory rate.
- And, yeah, not too much, if any, wine.

Infrared Light & Melatonin

While melatonin is most celebrated as a "sleep hormone," it double-agents as a powerful antioxidant.

An antioxidant is a substance that can prevent or slow damage to cells caused by free radicals, unruly molecules that the body makes as a product of energy creation and in reaction to environmental forces. When unchecked, free radicals badly damage cells and their mitochondria and cause oxidative stress.

Melatonin is a direct scavenger of free radicals and reactive oxygen species (ROS). This means it can neutralize these harmful substances and reduce oxidative stress, which is associated with aging and many chronic diseases, including cancer, neurodegenerative diseases, cardiovascular disease, and diabetes.

Melatonin is particularly effective in protecting mitochondria, the energy-producing parts of cells that are particularly vulnerable to damage from free radicals. Melatonin can also stimulate the activity of other antioxidant enzymes like glutathione in the body, enhancing the overall antioxidant defense system.

We are already aware that melatonin is the "hormone of darkness," secreted by the pineal gland at night. But free radicals don't just operate under the cover of night. They are wreaking plenty of daytime havoc. So, how does the body protect itself during the day?

It turns out that near-infrared radiation (NIR) from the sun directly activates the production of melatonin at the subcellular level.

You cannot see near-infrared radiation, which registers between 760 and 1400 nm on the wave spectrum, as it is outside the parameters of visible light. But your sensory neurons can feel it as warmth—even through a shirt. The longer low-frequency wavelengths of near-infrared radiation more easily penetrate objects, just like the low-end frequency waves of the sonic spectrum emanate out of gold-rimmed SUVs.

Infrared radiation penetrates down into your body's tissue up to eight centimeters into cells and even into your mitochondria. Why is this important?

Your mitochondria are the energy-producing organelles in your cells that generate the currency known as ATP. It accomplishes this through a series of highly complex operations. One of the stages of energy production (or cellular respiration) is called the Krebs cycle. One of the primary by-products of the Krebs cycle is NADH, packaged reduced electrons that subsequently zip around the inner membrane of the mitochondria. At the end of this electron chain, there is an enzyme that catalyzes a reaction in which leftover electrons combine with oxygen to form water. The responsible enzyme is cytochrome C-oxidase (CCO). Like hectic factories can sometimes produce defective products, the process of energy making doesn't always function to perfection, and free radicals like superoxide and hydrogen peroxide are made.

Near-infrared radiation penetrates the skin and reacts with CCO. This excitation stimulates the production of melatonin at the mitochondrial level! In fact, 95 percent of your melatonin is produced on-site in the mitochondria and is consumed locally to blunt the impacts of free radicals. The melatonin stimulated by light is subcellular and does not enter the bloodstream. By extension, it does not make you sleepy.

The good news is that most of the energy on Earth is in the infrared spectrum. And you don't need to be in the sun to get it. Near-infrared radiation is actually stronger when it's reflected off leaves or grass. Being outside in green spaces, even in the shade, will upregulate the production of melatonin and, in turn, decrease oxidative stress.

Parenthetically, while sunscreen blocks ultraviolet rays, it does not inhibit NIR radiation from penetrating your skin. Also, the trappings of urbanity like buildings, concrete, and hot dog stands do not reflect near-infrared radiation light.

This interplay between near-infrared radiation light and your mitochondria may be one of the primary reasons why people who spend more time in nature have significantly reduced risk of type 2 diabetes and cardiovascular disease as well as less stress and lower blood pressure. As if we needed yet another reason to be in nature.

UVB (or Not to B)

Ultraviolet B radiation is a double-edged sword. It has both beneficial and harmful effects on the body. Thus, finding the right balance of ultraviolet B is key to health.

UVB radiation stimulates the production of vitamin D in the skin. Vitamin D is also a hormone in that it controls how cells and organs function. Vitamin D is a crucial nutrient that has multiple roles in the body.

It is required to absorb calcium and phosphate from the gut into the bloodstream. These minerals are critical for the development and maintenance of healthy teeth and bones. Deficiency in vitamin D can lead to a softening of the bones, a condition known as rickets in children and osteomalacia in adults. Long-term deficiency can contribute to osteoporosis.

Vitamin D is also important for maintaining muscle function. Deficiency can lead to muscle weakness and falls, particularly in older adults.

Vitamin D helps to regulate the body's inflammatory response. Research suggests that vitamin D may play a role in preventing and treating a number of different conditions, including type 1 and type 2 diabetes, hypertension, glucose intolerance, and multiple sclerosis.

Exposure to sunlight, including UVB radiation, can help improve mood and alleviate symptoms of seasonal affective disorder. There's some evidence to suggest that vitamin D might play a role in mood regulation and may help to ward off depression.

Vitamin D plays a significant role in the immune system, affecting both the innate and adaptive immune responses. Here's a closer look at how vitamin D interacts with immune cells:

The "innate immune system" is the body's first line of defense against pathogens. Immune cells in this system, such as macrophages and dendritic cells, have vitamin D receptors. When these cells are exposed to pathogens, they can increase the expression of the enzyme required to convert the inactive form of vitamin D in the body (25-hydroxyvitamin D) into its active form. Once activated, vitamin D can stimulate the production of antimicrobial proteins that kill pathogens and reduce inflammation.

The "adaptive immune system" involves T cells and B cells that respond to specific antigens and have memory capabilities, meaning they can provide long-term protection against specific pathogens. Vitamin D can help to regulate the adaptive immune system, promoting a balance between different types of T cells. This can help to prevent overactive immune responses and reduce inflammation.

Vitamin D can also inhibit the proliferation of B cells (which produce antibodies) and reduce the production of pro-inflammatory cytokines, which are substances secreted by immune cells that can cause inflammation.

Vitamin D keeps the porridge of the immune system just right, enhancing the body's natural defenses against pathogens while preventing overactive immune responses that could lead to chronic inflammation and autoimmune diseases.

Most of us enjoy a day frolicking on the beach, sunbathing, and perhaps sipping a tropical drink from a bamboo tumbler, but there are some significant cons to getting too much UVB radiation.

Excessive exposure to UVB radiation increases the risk of skin cancer, including melanoma, the most dangerous type of skin cancer. UVB radiation also accelerates skin aging, leading to wrinkles, age spots, and loss of skin elasticity. UVB radiation can cause damage to the eyes, increasing the risk of conditions like cataracts and corneal sunburn. Yes, your eyes can get sunburned along with the rest of your body, where it can cause pain, skin peeling, and, in severe cases, blistering.

So, what is the proper amount of time to spend in the sun? Well, oddly, it's completely bio-individual and determined largely by how much melanin you have. Melanin is the pigment responsible for the color of the skin, hair, and eyes in humans.

It plays a critical role in protecting the skin from the harmful effects of ultraviolet radiation from the sun. However, melanin's protective property also influences the synthesis of vitamin D in the skin, which is triggered by exposure to UVB radiation from the sun.

Melanin absorbs UV radiation and dissipates it as heat, providing a natural protection against sunburn and skin cancer. The more melanin in the skin, the darker the skin color and the more protection there is against UV radiation.

While melanin's ability to absorb UV radiation protects the skin from damage, it also reduces the skin's capacity to produce vitamin D. When UVB rays hit the skin, they interact with a form of cholesterol in the skin, which starts the process of vitamin D synthesis. But if those UVB rays are absorbed by melanin, fewer of them are available to start the vitamin D production process. This means that individuals with darker skin, who have more melanin, are at a greater risk of vitamin D deficiency if they don't get enough sun exposure, don't consume enough vitamin D in their diet, or don't take a vitamin D supplement.

This is a prime example of the trade-offs in human biology. The advantage of having more melanin is greater natural protection against sun damage and skin cancer, but the disadvantage is a higher risk of vitamin D deficiency, particularly in regions with less sun exposure. Conversely, individuals with less melanin (lighter skin) can synthesize vitamin D more readily, but they are at higher risk of sunburn and skin cancer.

For example, if you have darker skin and live in a high-latitude climate, you will almost certainly be vitamin D deficient. Of course, humans co-evolved with their climates, so high concentrations of melanin, for example, in most of Africa or India was an adaptive advantage. However, through migration and other more nefarious means, the world has gotten a lot "smaller" and multi-ethnic. This has led to evolutionary mismatches.

Once again, it's a balance. The need for sun exposure to produce vitamin D versus the risk of skin damage from the sun. The UV index can serve as your beach time planner. You can test to determine where or not you have a vitamin D deficiency. Optimal levels fall between 50 and 100 ng/mL (nanograms per milliliter). Levels below 20 ng/mL are considered deficient. Fortunately, supplementation of vitamin D is easy and relatively cheap. The recommended maximum daily limit of vitamin D in healthy people is 4,000-5,000 IU.[5] That said, it's hard to overdose. Vitamin D toxicity, also called somewhat ridiculously hypervitaminosis D, is a very rare but potentially serious condition that occurs when you have excessive amounts of vitamin D in your body.

Humans are completely dependent on the sun. Without its electromagnetic energy, there would be no photosynthesis, and, by extension, no plant growth. And animals need plants for food and oxygen. Our last great extinction, 65 million years back, was caused by the Chicxulub meteor crashing into the Yucatan Peninsula. The impact triggered a nuclear winter that blocked the sun's rays and wiped out 80–90 percent of living species.[6]

Alongside this reliance, humans have also evolved with the sun. We developed adaptive mechanisms in relationship with our solar system's only star. Our circadian rhythm and our endogenous antioxidant and vitamin D production are examples of our evolutionary rapport with chemical reactions occurring 93 million miles away.

THE BODY IN BALANCE

Cortisol vs. Melatonin

Cortisol is a steroid hormone produced in the adrenal glands, and it's derived from cholesterol and insoluble in blood. It plays a significant role in maintaining your body's internal clock or circadian rhythm in tandem with its dance partner melatonin, its contraposing hormone.

Cortisol levels bottom out around midnight and rise naturally in the morning, triggering a flood of glucose that supplies an immediate energy source to your large muscles. This helps to get your sleepy head out of bed.

Cortisol levels decline across the course of the day, sometimes with mini peaks in the late afternoon. As I will explain in greater depth in the chapter about evolution and culture, cortisol is on a hormonal teeter-totter with melatonin. In a balanced system, melatonin secretion increases soon after the onset of darkness, eliciting a sensation of grogginess that propels you toward your pajama drawer and recumbency. Melatonin typically peaks in the middle of the night, between 2 A.M. and 4 A.M., and gradually dips during the second half of the night as cortisol is rising. Crests and troughs.

This tenuous hormonal balance is maintained by the suprachiasmatic nucleus, the central pacemaker of the circadian timing system. This internal clock, as described, is set by light, specifically blue light. Equilibrium between cortisol and melatonin is essential for maintaining the sleep-wake cycle.

A world of endless perceived threats, as depicted on the news or amplified by social media, can lead to the overproduction of cortisol. Chronic cortisol overload incites a variety of detrimental knock-on impacts including high blood sugar (which can lead to type 2 diabetes) and weight gain. Protracted elevated glucose levels provoke a vicious cycle of inflammation in the body.

High cortisol levels also injure the innate immune system and decrease the production of key immune cells like neutrophils and macrophages. This means chronic stress and its bedfellow cortisol will decrease your ability to fight off pathogens.

High cortisol levels can also disrupt the balance of healthy bacteria in your gut, which may lead to dysbiosis or intestinal permeability (leaky gut). This leads to endotoxemia, the flow of toxins into your bloodstream, which, in turn, activates the immune system's inflammatory response.

And elevated levels of cortisol can, of course, disrupt sleep, which is also essential for cognitive function, memory consolidation, autophagy, maintaining insulin sensitivity, and activating the glymphatic system that cleans out dysfunctional proteins (like beta-amyloid) that may lead to dementia.

Getting consistent good sleep is among the most important metrics of health. Quality sleep is reliant on balancing the yin of melatonin with the yang of cortisol.

CHAPTER 15

THE INATTENTION ECONOMY

Focusing the Mind

All of humanity's problems stem from man's inability to sit quietly in a room alone.

— Blaise Pascal

When I was struggling with my health, there were clear, objective metrics to which I could point. I was tipping the scale north of 200. My fasting blood glucose was hovering at 125 mg/dL. My lipid panels were lopsided with too many small, dense LDL particles and not enough high-density lipoproteins (HDL). In some ways, these signals were comforting, not because they were good, but because they were measurable. And what you can measure, you can improve.

But there was another aspect of my poor health that was more elusive in nature. I couldn't exactly put my thumb on it. It was subjective, not objective. I too often felt fidgety and distracted. I was prone to being easily agitated. I was particularly triggered by dunderhead "influencers" on social media, who, despite their vapidity, had 20 times the number of followers. I had difficulty maintaining a conversation without my mind drifting or, worse, checking my phone. I suppose my lack of focus could be reflected empirically in the number of books I read across the year 2017: zero!

I was hardly alone. The deluge of information incessantly surging at us is mismatched with our biology. Our brains aren't wired for the constant onslaught of pings, dings, and notifications. The "attention economy" is making us distracted, unfulfilled, and sick.

Distraction

Every August, Ffej set out in the sweltering summer heat to forage for figs. A mature fig tree can grow to 35 feet high and live for 200 years or more. They bear rough vibrant green deciduous leaves that are deeply lobed and exude a white milky latex when broken. An abundant tree will boast 300 figs.

In warm climes, figs mature in the late summer. When ripe, they feel soft and squishy, like a half-full water balloon. The sweet fig was in high demand on the savannah, and Ffej was fortunate and delighted to find a tree pregnant with fruit. Upon discovery, Ffej gathered the most accessible figs growing off branches at shoulder height, devouring many while also packing the balance in his satchel. After collecting the most readily available fruits, Ffej would move into the tree's interior and eventually climb its trunk to avail himself of the figs growing on higher branches. Ffej would not rest until he had denuded the tree of all its bounty. Then, to the great satisfaction of the tribe, Ffej returned to camp, belly full and loot in tow.

In my conversation with the neuroscientist Adam Gazalley, he constructed a wonderful metaphor that he dubs "information foraging" in which he compares the harvesting of figs with that of information.

Gazalley points out that, when fig trees are solitary, a forager such as Ffej will take his time to harvest all the fruit on the tree. However, if Ffej had come across a great grove of fig trees, his method for gathering would be quite different. He would harvest the most accessible figs off a tree, and then, noticing that a neighboring tree had more shoulder-high fruit, he would move on to that tree and, once again, collect the most readily available figs. Then he would notice yet another tree with glistening sweet figs begging to be picked. And off he would cavort to that tree. And this pattern would repeat itself.

The human mind is wired to follow new data as they appear. There are both neural, and in Ffej's case, caloric rewards associated with skipping to the next thing. The mind is subtly performing a cost-benefit analysis, attempting to determine how long one should stay at a particular tree before hopping to the next. If the next tree is quite far away, then one will stay put and gorge as many figs as possible from the current tree, even if there are eventually diminishing returns. But if the next tree is neighboring, then there is little incentive to stay.

This human proclivity related to fig foraging can be applied to information. Imagine it's Sunday and you've curled up with Melville's *Moby Dick*. You are likely to become engrossed in Ishmael's narrative of Ahab's maniacal quest of the whale that metabolized his leg. While you could put the book down and find another, there is little reward in doing so.

In today's culture, however, rarely do we have the opportunity to immerse ourselves in a novel. We consume information in short blips as we scroll. Articles are not read as part of a morning coffee and newspaper ritual. They are most generally scanned on a glowing screen. And, almost invariably, there is a link out of that article within its first paragraph or two. This architecture is by design as more clicks lead to more advertisement impressions, which, in turn, lead to more revenue for the publisher. The same way a forager is tempted by figs on a neighboring tree, a reader recognizes the diminishing returns of finishing the article. He's gotten the gist and clicks out. Of course, the new article also has a link or two within the first 100 words baiting the next click. And so on.

We switch and toggle. And toggle and switch. And who could blame us? If this proclivity has an avatar, it would be the ubiquitous logo of our favorite Cupertino-based tech company: an apple with a bite missing. In the palm of our hands, we hold the entirety of humanity's knowledge, a dubious trade-off for the inability to hold a thought.

We are model organisms in the mass human psychological experiment known as the attention economy. Every brand, agency, and influencer, not to mention parent, sibling, and child, are vying for your conscious attention at every possible second through pings and dings on text, e-mail, Slack, and multiple social media platforms.

This is on top of the quainter old-school methods like print ads, TV commercials, and billboards. Even planes fly by with banners trailing behind them, promoting all-you-can-eat buffet specials.

It is estimated that the average American checks their smartphone 352 times per day or once every three minutes, with 75 percent of us considering our phones a necessity rather than a luxury and 20 percent unwilling to go without it for more than a few hours. And another 75 percent of Americans tote it along regularly to the loo.[1]

My friend Jess Davis, founder of Folk Rebellion, hipped me to the term *nomophobia*. Yes, there's even a word for the fear of being without your phone or without cellular service.

What is the impact of the attention economy on our brains?

We have developed acute "monkey mind," where thoughts are branches and our minds are swinging riotously like chimps from one to another. Many of us are quite aware of this condition as a product of our own experience. Reading a book or sitting at the piano to figure out a song used to be easy and fulfilling activities for me. Now, I struggle to pursue my hobbies (and write this book) without checking my phone. I am undoubtedly not the exception.

In 2022, the group Words Rated surveyed 2,003 American adults in order to better understand the reading habits of Americans. More than half of American adults (51.57 percent) haven't read a full book in over a year, 22.01 percent of adults haven't read a book in over 3 years, and 10.83 percent haven't read a book in more than 10 years.[2] This would be an opportune moment to express my gratitude to you for reading this book.

Linda Stone, a former Apple consultant, coined the phrase "continuous partial attention."[3] By adopting 24-7 "always on" behavior, modern humans exist in a state of constant alertness, scanning the world for shiny or dangerous objects but never really giving our full attention to anyone or to anything. This traps us in our sympathetic nervous system with its concomitant stress hormones that over time undermine immune function, gut health, and stable blood sugar.

By analogy with computers, we believe we are multitasking, but in reality, we are just rapidly switching between different activities. While the human brain can manage multiple passive activities, like driving while listening to a podcast, it cannot concentrate on several simultaneous areas of focus.

The consequences of distraction are severe as it degrades our ability to hold information at a high level of resolution and diminishes productivity. According to a study from the University of California, Irvine, it takes an average of 23 minutes and 15 seconds to regain focus on a specific task after a distraction.[4]

Harvard psychologists Matthew A. Killingsworth and Daniel T. Gilbert published a paper in *Science* called "A Wandering Mind Is an Unhappy Mind." The title of this study certainly deviates from many of the more technically named papers published in the highly stringent journal. In their study, Killingsworth and Gilbert report that people spend 46.9 percent of their waking hours thinking about something other than what they're doing, and this mind-wandering typically makes them patently unhappy.[5]

"A human mind is a wandering mind, and a wandering mind is an unhappy mind," Killingsworth and Gilbert write. "The ability to think about what is not happening is a cognitive achievement that comes at an emotional cost."

Unlike our furry friends in the animal world, *Homo sapiens* spend voluminous hours thinking about what is not happening. We brood over the events of the past and project them into the future as "anticipated memories."

Even our more positive daydreaming appears to have a negative impact on happiness. We woolgather about tropical vacations, impending hot dates, and potential work promotions. But, all that time, we're not really here. And here—in the ever now—is the only place happiness can truly exist. You can't be happy in the future.

Ffej was habituated to a whole lot of nothing. Of course, there was a to-do list of biological imperatives. But there was no way to communicate except face-to-face. And there was no one selling anything. Thich Nhat Hahn famously exhorted, "When you wash the dishes, wash the dishes." Ffej didn't even have dishes. It was easier to be present, to yoke intention and action. There was no brooding feeling of time scarcity or fear of missing out.

Increasingly, humans are unable to manage boredom. We can't wait in line at the grocery store without scanning Instagram or wait for the light to turn green without answering a text. Our lives have become a mile-wide and an inch deep. We're fidgety and off somewhere else.

So . . . how many times did you check your phone while reading this section?

Amygdala Hijack

Ffej usually foraged alone, snacking over the course of the day upon vegan delights, and also bringing honey, berries, baobab fruit, tubers, and occasional wild game back to the tribe. During the wet season, the tribe's diet was predominantly vegetarian. The contribution of meat to the diet increased in the dry season, when wildebeest, warthogs, buffalo, and giraffes became concentrated around sources of water. During this time, Ffej was often joined by a fellow tribesman and spent entire nights lying in wait by waterholes, hoping to shoot animals that approach for a nighttime drink with poison-treated arrows.

Sapiens, however, were not the only species roaming the Serengeti hunting wild game. Lions, leopards, cheetahs, and jackals slinked through tall grasses, surveying the landscape for potential prey. Humans made sumptuous appetizers for this group. And odd-toed ungulates, though primarily herbivorous, were not always fond of human encroachment. Ffej did his best to remain low key and out of sight. However, from time to time, he would be startled by a rustle in the grass or in a moment of carelessness attract the attention of a potential predator.

When this occurred, Ffej experienced an instantaneous physiological transformation. Perceived threat triggered his hind brain, specifically a small almond-shaped cluster of neurons in the medial temporal lobe known as the amygdala. The amygdala is famously associated with "fight or flight," your body's involuntary response to external threat. It interfaces with the hypothalamus-pituitary-adrenal (HPA) axis, the major neuroendocrine system that controls reactions to stress. Activation of the HPA axis results in the secretion of cortisol (and epinephrine). Cortisol is a glucocorticoid, a steroid hormone made from cholesterol in the adrenal glands. In response to perceived threat, cortisol is secreted from the adrenals into the bloodstream. The discharge of cortisol causes respiratory and heart rate to increase, blood to move from the gut to muscles in the extremities and pupils to dilate. It instantaneously readies you for fight or flight.

This adaptive mechanism had great utility for Ffej on the Serengeti. Fortunately for Ffej and his tribe, these intense instances of stress were few and far between. Cortisol levels never remained too high for too long. Once the threat had passed, the body would naturally move back into homeostasis. Breathing would normalize and heart rate would decrease.

Despite the array of acute paleolithic stressors in his life, Ffej actually enjoyed quite a bit of leisure time. He took great joy in climbing to the summit of local peaks and staring out at the vast landscape. From time to time, Ffej would spot flocks of guinea fowl or quail flying east in distinct patterns. This phenomenon would indicate an impending storm. This is how Ffej got his news. In witnessing the migration, Ffej would descend back to basecamp and alert his tribe that a storm was looming.

Of course, modern humans are awash in information. The competition for our attention is so intense that it uses paleolithic techniques. Everything from the latest Kardashian drama to the most current political scandal is framed as a biological threat to trigger the same mechanisms that caused Ffej to run for cover.

Let's imagine you were served up the following video titled: ***Social Media Is an Endocrine DISRUPTOR!!!***

Would this title scandalize you? Do the ALL CAPS catch your eye? Maybe, this title is too obscure. How about . . . ***YouTube Is Giving You DIABETES!!!*** Would that get you to click and watch?

If I was smart, I'd hire a pale nose-ringed Zoomer to A/B test both titles to see which one best tickled the algorithm. And then, in the content, I'd explain how YouTube videos are designed to hijack your amygdala in the same manner that a charging rhino triggered Ffej's hind brain. This content is designed to send signals down your HPA axis that activates the production of cortisol. And with every new video, YouTube refills the IV bag of cortisol that chronically drips through your bloodstream, heightening glucose levels and activating the release of insulin from your pancreas until an excess of insulin leads to a resistance to itself. And then you have diabetes. And, of course, at the end, I'd push you to the next video!

I'm creating this imaginary scenario ironically to prove a point. However, it does not deviate much from our modern reality.

Unlike Ffej, we live in an era where time and attention are the most precious of life's commodities. We subsist within the persuasion economy, sometimes also dubbed the attention economy, in which every marketer, influencer, and news outlet is vying for our mind-share at every possible moment. Headlines and product ads come in the form of social media posts, notifications, texts, remarketing campaigns, banner ads, and on.

The persuasion economy relies on hyperbole and salaciousness to snatch your attention; 24-hour news and social media influencers use anecdotes to create plausibility, wrap them in sensationalist titling, lace them with editorial bias, and deploy them like missiles to scare and outrage you. They leverage the algorithm that rewards hype over nuance and yelling over conversation for the purposes of garnering influence and followers, increasing watch time and selling advertisements.

No one political party or news outlet has a monopoly on this type of villainy. Just today, I foraged a number of diverse sensationally titled videos and articles from my inbox:

- "What REALLY caused the Maui fires?" from comedian-cum-political commentator Russell Brand
- "Kids and Teens Are Dying, But Why?" from the Children's Health Defense
- "The World Is on the Brink of Catastrophic Warming!" from the Democratic Election Fund
- "Donald Trump Going to Jail?" from MSNBC
- And my favorite . . . "Snakes Falling from Ceiling of Lexington High School" from Fox News

The psychological and physiological result of the great nonconsensual experiment of social media is chronic stress. Beyond the aforementioned impacts of cortisol, the chronic infusion of this hormone has myriad knock-on consequences. These impacts are worthy of reiterating. Cortisol is a master hormone, and while it's utterly useful in the right proportion, its excess is central to many of society's most common conditions.

Chronic cortisol disrupts your gut microbiome. It reduces diversity in the microbiome and leads to increased intestinal permeability, breaking down the tight junctions in the epithelium that prevent toxins from entering the bloodstream. This barrier is but one cell thick. When it is broken down, undigested food and decrepit bacterial membranes called lipopolysaccharides cross into the bloodstream and trigger an immune response. This leads to chronic inflammation, food allergies, and a variety of gut diseases.

Numerous studies have also shown that people with chronically high cortisol levels have reduced immune function. In response to chronic cortisol, the body produces less neutrophils and macrophages. These cells are essential to the innate immune system that provides the body with general protection from pathogenic bacteria. Innate immune cells also contribute to tumor suppression. They engage in a process called phagocytosis in which they literally engulf and "eat" malignant cells.

Cortisol also spikes blood sugar levels. Over time, this stresses the pancreas to produce more and more insulin to get serum glucose out of the bloodstream into cells. Eventually, cells become insulin resistant. As previously described, this can lead to diabetes.

Further, when glucose is left to linger in the blood, it can become glycated and cause inflammation. It also gets converted to triglycerides and stored as visceral fat. This type of fat that clusters around your belly and organs stresses the heart as it requires the production of increasingly more blood vessels. Visceral fat is also pro-inflammatory. These adipocytes release inflammatory cytokines like interleukin-6, which further disrupts immune function and also can pock up arterial walls, leaving them more susceptible to the accumulation of plaques from small, low-density lipoproteins. This phenomenon leads to cardiovascular disease—the world's number one killer.

So, is social media killing you? Well, let's not get too melodramatic about it. But, over time, being in a state of amygdala hijack will not only erode your physiological health but also compromise your ability to leverage the prefrontal cortex, the brain's locus of reason and rationality.

Is it possible to completely eschew all media and get your weather report like Ffej, sitting atop a peak? Probably not. However, you can certainly unfollow the more egregious sensationalists.

Fortunately, there is also a 4,000-year-old protocol that addresses our inability to focus, our attachment to our egos, and our chronic amygdala overload and its accompanying stress hormones. When I mention this practice to my children, they roll their eyes and say, "Dad! Don't you dare say the word *meditation*." But I do anyway.

On Meditation

The earliest records of meditation come from the Indian subcontinent. The Vedas, ancient Indian scriptures written around 1500 B.C.E., allude to meditation practices. The Upanishads, philosophical texts that date from around 500 B.C.E. to 400 B.C.E., also detail meditation and its benefits.

Despite its ancient roots, the word *meditation* itself can carry some unfortunate "New Age" baggage. Imagery of wafting frankincense, Ouija boards, and crystal pujas may appear in your mind's eye. Didn't we all have that kooky, if loveable, basket-weaving aunt who used to chant kirtan naked in the tall grass? Or perhaps that's too autobiographical? Regardless, I am here to dispel the notion that you need to be a card-carrying hippie or commit to monasticism to excavate the nature of your mind.

You go to the gym to train your muscles. In some ways, you can consider meditation as the training of the mind. And, like you need to stress your muscles in order to strengthen them, mind-training can initially feel taxing and uncomfortable.

Certainly, cultivating a meditation practice can improve concentration, relieve anxiety and stress, assuage fear, and ameliorate sleep. It can attenuate the strength of the ego's grip. It contributes to your holistic well-being, reducing inflammation, aiding digestion, and bolstering immunity. Engaging with the practice long-term actually changes the physiology of the brain. Meditation has been shown to increase the cortical thickness or gray matter concentration of the hippocampus—the part of the brain responsible for memory and regulating emotions.

However, while the benefits are multifarious, this practice should not be undertaken in pursuit of achieving a list of personal goals. The primary purpose of meditation is to access the present moment. And, in regularly doing so, the beneficial outcomes will become self-evident. So, in this manner, the process is the product. As you sharpen your ability to pay attention moment to moment, you will notice how the practice gradually begins to punctuate your quotidian life.

The second that you begin to contemplate all the potential improvements meditation may usher into your life, you've lost the primary plot. You're living in the future. The point is, as Watts described, to "groove with the present moment"—similar to how a musician or a dancer becomes absorbed in their art. It's not about getting anywhere. When you focus on the destination, then meditation, and life in general, becomes a dismal chore. At its very best, meditation is about flowing with the river's current. It's about being all here, right now.

There is a common misconception that meditation is about turning off the spigot of thoughts. Certainly, many of us suffer from the "monkey mind" I described a few pages back, a state of being where thoughts are branches and our minds are swinging wildly from one to another. We have trouble focusing or just being quiet. The majority of us can't make it through a stoplight without fidgeting with our phones. We have become addicted to occupying the mind. Of course, the mind is very useful, but so is my hand—but I am not obsessed with using it every millisecond.

Meditation doesn't turn thoughts off as much as it enhances our ability to witness them as phenomena arising and subsiding in consciousness moment to moment. We begin to witness thoughts in the same way we perceive sound or light or shadow. They are transitory happenings, coming and going. A meditation practice also helps us observe difficult emotions as passing phenomena so that we don't fixate on them or identify with them. We acknowledge them as they appear and wave at them as they disappear.

In this sense, we are the sky. Thoughts, feelings, and sensations are clouds. We are the road. Emotions are the cars, bicycles, and pedestrians. We are the precondition for everything that appears in a field of awareness, the blackboard upon which life is etched.

Humans have a penchant for fixating on thoughts generated from past experience and projecting those thoughts into the future as what Daniel Kahneman calls "negative anticipated memories."[6] For example, we might think about something bad that happened the last time we went to the doctor. When drawing blood, the nurse couldn't locate the vein and we almost passed out. And then we spend our time awash in worry about our appointment next month. In this way, much of our suffering is a phantom of our own projection. Because, most of the time, right now, we are totally fine. Meditation helps to migrate us out of the narrative life of our torturous past and imagined future and into the experienced life of the present.

In his Yoga Sutras, Patanjali spells out the "purpose" of yoga. To be clear, Patanjali was writing about a very different kind of yoga than we are accustomed to in modern Western society. Modern yoga is primarily physical, derived from a branch of yoga known as Hatha yoga. There are postures—asanas—and physical sequences that move the practitioner between various postures. However, historically, asana is but one of yoga's eight limbs. The balance of the limbs addresses ethics, meditation, and concentration. For all intents and purposes, Patanjali was primarily describing meditation in his yoga sutras. In the second verse, Patanjali lays out meditation's target with this simple phrase: *yogas chitta vritti nirodha*.[7]

Here's the rough translation from the Sanskrit:

> Yogas: yoga is
> Chitta: the mind
> Vritti: turning or fluctuating
> Nirodha: ceasing

Yoga is the ceasing of the turning of the mind. Or, more poetically, *yoga is the progressive stilling of the fluctuations of the mind*.

The Sanskrit meaning of the word *yoga* is to "yoke" or unite. By calming our incessant mental chatter, we can begin to yoke—cultivating a natural union within ourselves and between ourselves and the universe. As you become immersed in the present moment, eventually the subject-object dichotomy that pits you as separate from the world around you begins to dissipate. This is a glimpse into the mystical terminus of meditation. Samadhi, or integrated consciousness, is a state of nondualism at the end of the spiritual rainbow where the conventional notion of self dissolves and there is just the world.

Single Pointedness of Mind

As I have detailed, I was pulled a thousand different directions with pings and dings from notifications and texts and social media. Technology has degraded our concentration spans.

While meditation should not be undertaken to accomplish a list of goals, the ability to focus one's attention is one of the most useful by-products of this practice. The aptitude to cultivate long-wave thoughts not only helps you get things done but also builds discernment—the capacity to reason and delineate between fact and fiction, which is no simple task in the current environment. In many ways, meditation is a tuning fork for the truth.

Similar to how we build our biceps or abdominals, we can also train the muscle of our mind to focus. In Buddhism, there is the concept of dhāranā. In Chinese, this translates as *chan* and in Japanese as *zen*. Dhāranā can be understood as "concentration," but a better translation may be "single pointedness of mind."

The practice involves focusing on a distinct specific point. This could be a visual gaze point, known as a *kasina*. You find a comfortable seat and concentrate your conscious attention on a singular spot or location. Traditionally, the kasina are colors or the elements such as a rock, a pool of water, candle flame, light, or even space.

This focused gazing is known as *drishti*. Your focus point could also be a mandala or a yantra, but it could just as well be a coffee mug or the tip of your nose. The objective is to hold your attention. At some point, your focus will unavoidably waver. In this case, distraction is actually an opportunity to reset your concentration.

In their aforementioned paper, "A Wandering Mind Is an Unhappy Mind," Daniel Gilbert and Matthew Killingsworth speak to the inevitability of drifting attention. Here's the interesting bit. The "happiest" people turn out to be those who can most quickly return to their focus after being distracted.[8] The average time duration of refocusing your attention provides a potent gauge for progress.

A drishti need not necessarily be a visual point of focus. You can practice with a sonic drishti, sometimes known as a mantra, in which you repeat a phrase over and again. In some meditation traditions, you are given your own personal mantra. You can also just invent one.

Some 15 years ago, I was fortunate enough to tour with the jazz piano legend Herbie Hancock. Prior to every concert, I was invited into his inner backstage sanctum to chant. Herbie is a practicing Buddhist from the Nichiren school. The mantra *Nam Myōhō Renge Kyō* is a common Japanese chant within all forms of Nichiren Buddhism. In English, the words mean "Devotion to the mystic Law of the Lotus Sutra" or "Glory to the Dharma of the Lotus Sutra."

However, after 15 minutes of deep, resonant chanting, the words cease to mean anything at all. They just become vibrations. In a way, mantras are a gimmick, a tool that help us move into trans conceptual space, where we let go of symbols, words, and abstractions and connect to the substrate of reality. We're simply inhabiting the moment.

There are other ways to cultivate single pointedness of mind. Tibetan bowls, for example, can be used as sonic points of focus. Essential oils, incense, and other olfactory stimuli can be leveraged as tools to foster focus. Mala beads threaded between the thumb and index finger offer a way to take note of the cycles of inhalation and exhalation. There are 108 malas (beads) on a sutra (thread). The length of a meditation session can be regulated by how long it takes to go around the necklace, with each bead representing an inhale and exhale.

Practicing single pointedness of mind is initially very difficult and frustrating. It quickly reveals the monkey mind. However, with practice, you become more adept at returning to your focus when you lose it. Once this conscious effort becomes subconscious, you will begin to notice how much easier it is to concentrate, read a book . . . or even write one.

The Breath

Of course, the breath can also serve as a potent point of singular focus. Different patterns of inhalation (always through the nose), holds, and exhalation provide our conscious attention with a place to anchor our awareness. The breath is always with us—I suppose, until it isn't—but while we are occupying this physical plane, the breath is always at our disposal.

Generally, breathing is governed by the autonomic nervous system. In other words, day-to-day, it functions completely below the crust of consciousness as a bottom-up behavior. However, it is the one component of the autonomic nervous system over which we have conscious agency. And, in this way, the breath is a conduit to the subconscious. As thoughts, emotions, and sensations appear in awareness, sometimes pulling us into mental busyness, we can always return to the presence and rhythm of the breath.

Anapanasati is the meditation technique expressly taught by the Buddha as a tool for full awakening. The practice, which has its provenance in the Anapanasati Sutta, uses conscious breathwork to calm and focus the mind such that it is equipped to "see" into itself and let go into freedom.[9]

The initial step is to make your breath your exclusive object of attention, focusing on all the sensations produced in your nostrils, chest, lungs, and abdomen. As your breath awareness matures, this attention can be expanded to the entire body.

The Buddha wrote, "Being sensitive to the whole body, the yogi breathes in; being sensitive to the whole body, the yogi breathes out."[10]

Inevitably, phenomena—feelings, thoughts, emotions—will arise in awareness and take you off course. This is a chance to witness them without judgment, wave serenely at them as they subside, and simply return to the breath.

The Breath & Stress Response

We are aware of the two primary subdivisions of the autonomic nervous system: the sympathetic and the parasympathetic. We know that the sympathetic nervous system is associated with increased respiratory and heart rate and is concomitant with certain neuromodulators like epinephrine and cortisol. And, on the contrary, the parasympathetic nervous system is associated with decreased respiratory and heart rate and connected to more inhibitory neuromodulators like GABA and oxytocin.

Generally, this system operates automatically—hence its name. However, conscious breath is a tool we can use to render that which is generally unconscious conscious. For example, by purposefully slowing breath rate, you can move your body into a parasympathetic state. At the same time, by engaging in vigorous conscious breathwork, you can trigger the sympathetic system.

For example, the Wim Hof method is a breathing technique that upregulates the nervous system.It involves controlled hyperventilation in which you take in 30–50 forceful breaths. You breathe in fully but exhale only partially. The idea is to "overbreathe," and this triggers your sympathetic nervous system. After the repeated deep breathing, you exhale fully and then hold your breath for as long as you comfortably can. Your previous overbreathing dropped your CO_2 levels below normal, and this is the reason most people can hold their breath for much longer than usual. When you feel a strong urge to breathe, you take a recovery breath by inhaling and holding full for about 15 seconds, then exhale. This cycle is typically repeated for three to four rounds.[11]

This deliberate overbreathing method results in varying degrees of hypocapnia, lower than normal concentrations of CO_2 in your blood, which causes temporary blood alkalinity. The breath holding after the overbreathing often results in hypoxia (low oxygen levels in the blood). From a neuromodulator and hormonal perspective, the overbreathing often induces the secretion of cortisol and adrenaline. This is advantageous if it's deliberate. For example, if you are in a situation where you want to be alert, this technique will trigger the molecules that will make you feel attentive and on the ball.

On the other hand, perhaps you are looking for relief from a stressful situation or extreme anxiety. In this case, overbreathing would not be recommended. Instead you will want to consciously leverage the breath to induce a parasympathetic state. You purposefully decrease respiratory rate which will bring down heart rate and blunt excitatory neuromodulators. Popular parasympathetic-inducing techniques include extending your exhalations as well as box breathing or Andrew Weil's 4-7-8 breathing pattern.

The box breathing technique consists of a four-count inhale, a four-count hold, a four-count exhale, and a four-count hold. And repeat. The 4-7-8 praxis consists of a four-count inhale, a seven-count hold, and an eight-count exhale. In both cases, breathe lightly and slowly. Both of these techniques induce a rest and digest state and are very effective for reducing anxiety and going to sleep.

Both meditation and breathwork are highly effective stress management tools. In a world that rewards the leveraging of fear and anger, these practices help to move you back into the rational neo-mammalian brain.

As the body preps for fight or flight in reaction to a new startling piece of information, there is a simultaneous, countervailing action that emerges in the hippocampus, the brain region dedicated to memory storage, threat perception, and the fear mitigation response. Along with the prefrontal cortex, the rational decision-making part of the brain, these centers of reason assess the legitimacy of a threat. If the hippocampus and prefrontal cortex decide that the fear response is exaggerated, they can dampen the amygdala's activity.

Again, let us remember Frankl's famous axiom, "Between stimulus and response there is a space. In that space is our power to choose our response. In our response lies our growth and our freedom."

Meditation and breathwork cultivate that space.

Deliberate Hypoxia

The breath, or lack of it, can also be leveraged consciously for physiological benefit.

If you want to train like an Olympian, then you might consider a trip to Colorado Springs, Mammoth Lakes, or Flagstaff. You wouldn't be going for the local cuisine or the nightlife. You'd book a ticket for the thin air. All these locations boast top-notch training facilities and share an elevation between 6,000 and 8,000 feet above sea level.

It's not that the concentration of oxygen in the atmosphere is any less at higher altitude, but the atmospheric pressure drops. At sea level, the atmospheric pressure is approximately 760 millimeters of mercury, and the concentration of oxygen in the air is about 20.9 percent. As altitude increases, atmospheric pressure decreases. At 6,000 feet above sea level, the atmospheric pressure drops to roughly 633 mmHg, which reduces the partial pressure of oxygen. This reduction in partial pressure leads to a decrease in the amount of oxygen available for the body to use, which can lead to a condition known as hypoxia.

Severe hypoxia can induce loss of consciousness, organ damage, and even death. Chronic hypoxia can cause hypertension. You definitely do NOT want respiratory or circulatory hypoxia (also known as ischemia), which is caused by inadequate blow flood to tissues. But deliberate *environmental* hypoxia in the right dose can be a good stress.

Deliberate or controlled hypoxia is the practice of intentionally exposing oneself to lower levels of oxygen either through training at high altitudes, specific breathing techniques, or using hypoxic training devices. There are breath-holding exercises, like the previously described Wim Hof method, that temporarily reduce the oxygen available to the body, inducing a mild hypoxic state. There are also hypoxic air machines, masks, and chambers that generate air with reduced oxygen content which is then inhaled.

The potential benefits of controlled hypoxia are pleiotropic. More generally, when exposed to "good" stressors in the right dosage, the body adapts. By extension, adaptation to intermittent hypoxia leads to more efficient use of oxygen.

More specifically, hypoxia stimulates the production of erythropoietin (EPO) by the kidneys, leading to an increased production of red blood cells and improved oxygen delivery to muscles. This results in enhanced endurance and athletic performance due to better oxygen utilization. Hypoxic training can promote mitochondrial biogenesis (the creation of new mitochondria), improve the efficiency of existing mitochondria, and create a shift toward more fat utilization for energy. Hypoxia can induce the production of vascular endothelial growth factor (VEGF), a signal protein that promotes the growth of new blood vessels. This leads to improved blood supply to various tissues, including muscles, which can aid in recovery and performance.

Additionally, some studies suggest that intermittent hypoxia can improve insulin sensitivity and glucose metabolism and, by extension, prevent type 2 diabetes. Controlled hypoxia can improve the balance between the sympathetic and parasympathetic branches of the autonomic nervous system. This can lead to better heart rate variability and a better stress response.

Letting Go

There is also a mystical aspect to meditation and breathwork. As your practice deepens, the feeling of being a separate ego-self begins to dissipate.

In fact, the ultimate target of the practice is the unwinding of the ego. You cease identifying with what you have and what others think of you. You stop craving, clinging, and comparing. You begin to feel a greater sense of connection and interdependence with the world. In Buddhism, this is known as *samadhi*, the transformation in consciousness from being an isolated self to the sensation of being completely integrated with the universe.

Instead of feeling jealous of another person's accomplishments, you might feel what the Buddhists call "mudita"—or joy simply for someone else's joy. You might cultivate greater compassion (karuna) where you identify the suffering of others as your own.

The translation of *nirvana* is literally "to blow out." To exhale. To let go. To forgive. To stop clinging to your ego, to remove the many cloaks of identity you've layered on. Letting go is the work of a lifetime. And a lifetime begins and ends with a breath.

THE BODY IN BALANCE

The Nervous System

The nervous system is the part of you that coordinates action and sensory information through the transmission of myriad signals to and from the body.

The nervous system is made up of the central nervous system—the brain and spinal cord—and the peripheral nervous system—neurons that branch off from the spinal cord and extend to all parts of the body.

Top Down vs. Bottom Up

The peripheral nervous system also has two subsystems: the somatic nervous system and the autonomic nervous system.

These systems relate to two different kinds of physiological and psychological behavior. The somatic system includes functions that are under your conscious control, like the voluntary movement of your muscles. This kind of intentional and deliberate action is known as top-down behavior. You are strolling down the aisles of a market, looking for radishes. There's a glorious bunch of them in a bin, and you consciously reach down, grab them, and nestle them snugly in your cart. This action, prosaic though it may be, exemplifies the top-down behavior associated with the somatic system, which also helps you process the senses of touch, sound, taste, and smell.

Modern science, however, estimates that 97 percent of all human function occurs below the crust of consciousness as involuntary bottom-up behavior.[12] Respiration, cardiac function, digestion and metabolism, immune function, and detoxification are among the many unconscious functions of the body. Further, emotions like fear and love, anger and compassion, envy and tranquility depend on the 97 percent of brain activity that lies underneath conscious awareness.

These subconscious processes are the province of the autonomic nervous system, the part of your overall nervous system that controls the "automatic" functions of your body that you need to survive.

It may be no surprise that the autonomic nervous system also has yang-yin subsystems: the sympathetic and parasympathetic systems.

As a means of understanding these contrapuntal systems, let's take a brief foray into the neurobiology of fear. Fright is a product of the brain and mediated by our autonomic nervous system, which regulates bodily functions such as heart rate, digestion, respiratory rate, pupillary response, urination, and sexual arousal. This system functions autonomously, hence its name: below the crust of conscious effort. The autonomic nervous system has two primary divisions: the parasympathetic and the sympathetic. The parasympathetic nervous system is most associated with "rest and digest," decreasing respiration and heart rate and increasing gastrointestinal activity. The sympathetic nervous system directs the body's rapid involuntary response to dangerous or stressful situations. A flash flood of hormones boosts the body's alertness and heart rate, sending extra blood to the muscles. How does this work, exactly?

The "fight, flight, or freeze" response is initiated in a region of the brain called the amygdala. This almond-shaped mass of neurons in the temporal lobe is dedicated to detecting the emotional salience of stimuli. A threat, such as the sight of a drunken man running toward you with a chainsaw, triggers a fear reaction in the amygdala, which in turn, activates neural areas responsible for motor functions relating to either putting up a fight, getting the hell out of Dodge, or becoming a possum.

What ensues is an internal neural debate between fear and reason (as if there could be any deliberation more emblematic of our times).

The amygdala interfaces with the endocrine system via the hypothalamus. The hormones epinephrine and cortisol are secreted into the bloodstream, leading to a rise in blood pressure and pulmonary activity and a reduction of commotion in the stomach and intestines. Glucose is shuttled to your muscle while pupils dilate and vision becomes tunneled.

While the body preps for fight or flight, there is a simultaneous, countervailing action that emerges in the hippocampus, the brain region dedicated to memory storage, that mitigates the fear response. Along with the prefrontal cortex, the rational decision-making part of the brain, these centers of reason assess the legitimacy of a threat. If the hippocampus and prefrontal cortex decide that the fear response is exaggerated, they can dampen the amygdala's activity. For example, if the raging man with the chainsaw is simply being projected on a movie screen, our sensible "thinking brains" will overpower the primal parts of the brain's automated fear response.

Both the sympathetic and parasympathetic systems have utility. The sympathetic system is essential for the biological imperative to survive. It allows the body to instantaneously respond to perceived threat. The parasympathetic system is crucial for healthy digestion and immune system balance.

The key to psychological well-being is a healthy balance between the sympathetic and parasympathetic systems, and, particularly, between the hormones that are concomitant with each system. Unfortunately, our modern culture contributes to sympathetic overload, a state that induces the chronic secretion of the stress hormone cortisol.

Across years of information excess and overwork, my nervous system had been clearly "yanged." I, like so many others, suffered from amygdala hijack. The incessant flood of fear-based news and social media sensationalism kept its foot on the cortisol pedal. And too much chronic cortisol led to high serum glucose levels, gut dysbiosis, and immune system imbalance. By incorporating meditation and conscious breath, I brought both my psychological and physiological health into greater equilibrium.

CHAPTER 16

STRESSFUL CONVERSATIONS

Eating Dirt & Leaning In

What does it mean to be insulted? Stand by a stone and insult it, what response will you get? Likewise, if you listen like a stone, what would the abuser gain by his abuse? However, if you have some weakness, then he has an advantage over you.

— EPICTETUS, *DISCOURSES*, 1.25

"How much is Pfizer paying you?"

"Another white man centering himself. . . PATHETIC!"

"Libtard!!!"

And more succinctly . . . "You're a dick! Unsubscribe."

These messages are but a small sampling of the hundreds of invidious e-mails that I received during the summer of 2020. Let me explain.

In March of that fateful year, as we anchored into Port Lockdown, I began writing a regular Sunday newsletter titled *Commusings*. My business partner, Jake, convinced me that these weekly essays could serve as buoys of hope for people navigating the choppy seas of COVID-19. Indeed, words can be vessels for emotions and, when we share them, we can feel less alone. Naively, I agreed to the task.

However, before too long, I found myself over a literary barrel every Saturday, pressured to produce 2,000 words of sense-making at a time when little made sense.

Fortunately for my column (and unfortunately for much of the world), 2020 offered plenty of putrid fodder about which to write. In addition to our wicked global pandemic, there was the murder of George Floyd and the ensuing national reckoning around social justice. There was, of course, the presidential election, the rise of QAnon, and countless other seismic rumblings emanating out of Trumplandia.

Social media is a wonderful tool for sharing family photos, but it is an awful sandbox for public discourse. Anyone who spends time on the Serengeti of Twitter (now X) or Facebook is aware of the vitriol, the strawmanning, and the ad hominem attacks. I decided to take a decidedly different course. I chose to pen long-form essays grounded in rigorous research, multiple perspectives, and humor where it was available. Perhaps foolishly, I attached my personal e-mail to these screeds, which were sent to over a million souls scattered around the globe.

As a result of this project, I received an unexpected lesson in building my psychological resilience.

When I awoke each Monday morning, a deluge of incoming e-mails flooded my inbox. Many of these messages were supportive and thankful, but hundreds were not. On the contrary, they were brimming with expletives and personal attacks. Across 2,000 words, my *Commusings* offered plenty of opportunity to offend. There always seemed to be one idea or turn of phrase that didn't sit right with someone.

I got criticism from all sides of the sociopolitical spectrum. Apparently, I was simultaneously an officer of the woke police *and* a racist colonizer. I was charged with being at once a shill for pharma *and* a science-denier. I was accused of being both a radical leftist *and* a limp incrementalist.

I wrote one lengthy article about COVID that I published in August of 2020. My research clearly suggested that people with comorbidities—specifically diabetes and obesity—were disproportionately impacted by the virus. According to the data, those who suffered from these chronic conditions were significantly more likely to contract severe cases of the disease. This finding was clearly reflected in hospitalization and fatality statistics. In the essay, I made great efforts to separate the health dimensions of obesity from its cultural aspects. Still, many people felt as if I was "fat-shaming" them, and they didn't hesitate to let me know in quite brutal fashion.

Of course, as someone who had struggled with weight, I presumed that readers would understand that I was speaking directly to the health implications of obesity. I assumed incorrectly. Initially, I took the criticism very personally. I was defensive. I was simply trying to write a thoughtful free newsletter. I felt hurt and spent many a night brooding over my rejoinders, holding the embers of revenge and plotting the right moment to hurl them. Of course, all that time, it was me who was getting burned.

Despite my initial defensiveness, over the course of the summer, I slowly built what my dearest Schuyler dubs my *psychological immune system*.

Schuyler contends that she rarely falls ill because, as a kid, she ate so much dirt. If you were to visit her childhood home (still inhabited by her hippie parents), you would accept her claim with little argument. Long-forgotten dust bunnies garnish the creaky floorboards, and elaborate cobwebs ornament the rafters. I am sneezing just writing about it.

If you tried to bounce a dime on the bed sheets, it would likely vanish into the black hole of a crusty paisley comforter from the '80s. The abundance of love radiating through that old wooden house is matched only by the utter dearth of cleaning products.

While the house had its grubby charms, Schuyler is mostly referring to the immense amount of time she spent outdoors, tripping around her mom's vast vegetable garden, collecting worms, and building tree forts.

While the copious consumption of dirt in and of itself might not ward off disease, Schuyler's ingestion of the bounteous microbes that reveled in the bacterial bordello that was her home may well have contributed to her sturdy constitution.

Indeed, there is increasing evidence from scientific studies that support the "hygiene hypothesis." This theory posits that disease, especially autoimmune conditions, are more common in the "developed" world because of the prevalence of antibacterials (and antibiotics) that reduce children's contact with microbes.

In short, one builds one's biological immune system through low-grade exposure to bacteria and viruses. Of course, many vaccines leverage this very mechanism. The chickenpox vaccine, for example, contains an attenuated virus that gives its recipient a diminutive viral load. In turn, the body produces antibodies that are subsequently on call to fight off a naturally occurring varicella viral infection. As I learned, a similar mechanism can be leveraged to produce "psychological antibodies."

Psychological Resilience

The great Stoics argued that you can develop your *psychological* immune system in much the same way you build physiological immunity. Fortunately, the wonderful British philosopher Jules Evans introduced me to Stoicism, a philosophy of personal ethics founded by Zeno of Citium in the 3rd century B.C.E.

Stoicism celebrates the development of resilience through subjection to adversity. Now, to be clear, this theory in no way justifies abuse, neglect, or other odious behavior that can induce trauma. However, Stoicism posits that the optimal way to disarm an insult is to be unaffected by it.

Exposure to insult and ridicule builds up mental resilience such that, on the face of it, one becomes indifferent—like being exposed to the chickenpox virus while possessing immunity. The ancient Greeks dubbed this quality of character *euthymia*, a state of unflappable positivity that emerges from living calmly and steadily and being undisturbed by fear or offense.

The celebrated Stoic and emperor of Rome, Marcus Aurelius, wrote, "Be like the rock that the waves keep crashing over. It stands unmoved and the raging of the sea falls still around it."

The practice of Stoicism also helped me to cultivate compassion as it offers the opportunity for cognitive reappraisal. When receiving a mean-spirited message, I would pause and ask myself, "What are the conditions in someone's life that would lead them to write me such a vindictive e-mail?"

I began to develop a greater compassion for people's short fuses. The entire world was at a boiling point, and people were sheltered in place, feeling isolated. Some degree of odious behavior was comprehensible. By the late summer of 2020, I began to look forward to negative feedback as a psychological challenge. I would eagerly await the Good Stress of moral censure to crest the bow of my inbox. And, inevitably, it did.

Upon receipt of disparagement, instead of harboring anger or countering with my own barb, I would kindly invite my more thoughtful detractors to join me on a Zoom call. This offer flummoxed most folks into retreat. In fact, sometimes I refer to this as my David Copperfield routine, as I made many of my hecklers disappear. However, approximately two dozen brave souls took me up on my offer.

During August and September 2020, I set aside Monday and Tuesday afternoons to have hour-long video calls with people that didn't agree with me.

I didn't initially have any training in empathic communication. I was operating by instinct. Relatively quickly, I noticed that these thorny conversations began to take on a distinguishable pattern. My antagonist and I would enter the virtual "room," jab at buttons for a moment, and then engage in some introductory pleasantries. As soon as we were two-dimensionally face-to-face, tempers were tempered and daggers dulled. The tone, even on Zoom, was completely different than on e-mail. After some hellos, I let them speak. And speak and speak and speak, they did.

Over and again, people just prattled on about their annoying bosses, their horrible-adorable children, their aching backs, and their aging cocker spaniels. They told me their life stories until, after 45 minutes or so, they had exhausted themselves.

I got better at these calls over time. I scribbled notes as people blathered, logging areas where our life experiences overlapped. And, finally, when I did speak, I would focus on those areas of convergence. My rejoinders included prosaic areas of coincidence such as:

"I also drove cross-country, and my car broke down."

"I also have three daughters."

"I was born in Chicago too."

Eventually, I learned from my friend and teacher John Kinyon that this technique reflected one of the core principles of nonviolent communication: seek connection before solution.

Nonviolent communication (a.k.a. NVC) is a communication system developed by psychologist Marshall Rosenberg that focuses on empathy, compassionate listening, and honest self-expression.

The primary goal of NVC is to connect at a human level and understand each other's needs. Finding solutions or agreements is secondary to establishing mutual understanding and empathy.

In my Zoom conversations, my guest and I would sometimes get around to discussing the initial issue that had put us at loggerheads. But, many times, we never did. It's hard to hate up close. Mostly, I learned that people just wanted to be seen and be heard.

After two months, I had made a bunch of new *frenemies*—from hard-core Trumpers to those wanting to abolish the police—and, along the way, I built my temperamental immunity. Before my summer of stressful conversations, I was psychologically brittle and unstable. It didn't take much to throw me off-center. Now I'm more of a weeble-wobble. I would weeble, but I wouldn't fall down. Psychological stress helped me develop equanimity, balance, and the ability to come back to center.

Emotional Resilience & Hard Conversations

Of course, Ffej never had any "virtual" conversations. It's not that he never was faced with disagreements and tense conversations, but he had little choice but to confront these challenges directly and face-to-face. We now live in a world of digital warriors waging battles anonymously from behind keyboards. People feel the liberty to be mean-spirited without the accountability of true, honest confrontation. There always seems to be someone cutting you down to size, doubting your abilities, or belittling your opinions.

Our modern invective offers two choices. These options are intriguingly mirrored in Brazilian jiujitsu, a martial art that deals with conflict through managing space. As master blackbelts Rener and Ryron Gracie taught me, the best way to get severely injured is to stand right where an assailant can step in and leverage all their body weight to punch you in the nose. If you step back, an attacker cannot connect. If you move in, they flail away with no clout and eventually collapse in exhaustion.

This physical tactic is also applicable to managing verbal conflict. It provides you with two options for remaining emotionally stable in response to an attack.

Option 1: You can disengage with the "virtual" world, shut off digital media, and focus on local and in-person relationships. You can also simply disregard insult. This is the equivalent of walking away from a fight. You just let the haters hate.

Option 2: You can lean in. If you choose to actively engage in thorny "stressful" conversations, and there's every reason in the world to do so, then first you must cultivate your own equipoise.

If you are in a state of hyperarousal, your ability to connect and have rational conversation will be impaired. In hyperarousal, you react as if you are under threat. You see the world as untrustworthy and menacing.

On the other hand, "bad" stress and trauma can elicit a state of hypoarousal also known as the dorsal vagal response. This response occurs when the body perceives extreme danger that it deems inescapable. It is a shutdown state that can manifest in dissociation and emotional numbing.

Both hyperarousal and hypoarousal impede attunement, the ability to connect authentically with the world. In his book *Attuned*, Austrian author Thomas Hübl also calls this state heart coherence.[1] When we cultivate euthymia and stillness, we foster the capacity for greater coherence and connection. We stop perceiving the world, even our aggressors, as threats. We refine our powers of perception and align our energy fields with those around us.

There are two steps required to host fruitful, hard conversations. The first involves your own personal development. The second consists of developing techniques for effective engagement.

Step 1: Focus on the development of euthymia, a state of unflappable positivity that is undisturbed by fear or offense through the following concepts and techniques:

- Practice stillness. Be the rock that the world's waves crash over. Just sit and witness the world around you without judgment.
- Recognize that insults arise from the anger of the person delivering them. Don't make their rage your own.
- Douse the flames of anger with buckets of kindness and humor.
- Pause and examine the ground conditions that would lead someone to make an injurious comment.
- Welcome insult as an opportunity to build resilience and foster emotional balance.

Remember the best strategy for disarming an insult is to be unaffected by it. Someone may attempt to belittle you or convince you that you are inadequate. If you let it slide right off of you, you pilfer their power. And, in their impotency, they will have little choice but to cease their behavior. Remember the words of Seneca who wrote, "To bear trials with a calm mind robs misfortune of its strength and burden."

If you seek a state of internal calm and contentment, if you aspire to be resilient in the face of adversity, if you are searching for an opportunity for personal growth, consider the lesson I took from Schuyler's childhood: don't be afraid to eat a little dirt.

Step 2: Once you have fostered your own euthymia, then you can engage in "stressful" conversations leveraging these NVC-derived principles:

- Schedule your conversations (or they likely won't happen).
- Set and setting matter: create a safe and secure space for people to be heard and seen.

- Separate observations from evaluations, focusing on establishing facts without judgment.
- Share your feelings without being accusatory. And hear someone else's feelings without being defensive.
- Listen to understand, not to respond: don't focus on forming rebuttals while the other person is speaking.
- Identify needs and make clear requests: articulate clearly what need is being unmet and how this need would be met.
- Seek connection, not solution: find areas of common ground even if agreement is not possible.

If we can have stressful conversations with people we barely know, think of how useful this skill can be when applied to your most important relationships. The skills I learned engaging with strangers in 2020 led me to having honest, sometimes tricky, conversations with my family.

Having thorny conversations can be incredibly difficult. It's tempting to avoid them. But, in the end, it's Good Stress, as it is often these very conversations that stand between us and a more cooperative, compassionate world.

Steelmanning: A Great Technique for Stressful Conversations

One of the best techniques for finding areas of common ground when having stressful conversations is called steelmanning. The term originates from its opposite, more popularly used technique, "strawmanning." Strawmanning and steelmanning are two contrasting argumentative techniques that people leverage in discussions and debates.

Strawmanning involves misrepresenting or oversimplifying someone else's argument to make it easier to refute. This is done by creating a "straw man" version of the argument, which is weaker or more extreme than the original, and then attacking this feeble version rather than engaging with the actual argument presented. This technique is used because it's quite easy to knock down a man of straw.

Here's an example of a straw man argument between Madison and Adam focused on the politically divisive topic of renewable energy.

Madison argues: "Given the environmental impacts of fossil fuels, we should invest more in renewable sources like solar and wind power to meet our energy needs."

Adam responds with a straw man argument by misrepresenting Madison's position, saying:

"Madison wants to shut down all coal and oil power plants immediately, leaving us without reliable energy on cloudy and windless days. That's an impractical and extreme position that would lead to widespread power outages and economic chaos."

In this example, Adam has distorted Madison's argument. Poor Madison was simply advocating for increased investment in renewable energy, not an immediate and complete switch from fossil fuels to renewables. By exaggerating and misrepresenting Madison's stance, Adam has transformed her into a straw man and then knocked her down, diverting the discussion away from the original, more nuanced argument about gradually increasing the use of renewable energy sources.

Steelmanning, on the other hand, represents the opposite approach. It involves echoing the best aspects of your opponent's argument. In our example, instead of issuing a rebuttal, Adam would first listen carefully to Madison's position and then reiterate the most compelling parts of it.

The goal of steelmanning is to engage with the best, most rational version of the opposing view. This approach promotes a more constructive and understanding dialogue. It fosters mutual respect, improves critical thinking, and facilitates genuine understanding. It helps ensure that disagreements are based on actual differences of opinion or values, rather than misunderstandings or misrepresentations of each other's views. Further, by addressing the strongest version of an opposing argument, you can fortify your own position and make it more resilient to criticism.

If Adam were to steelman Madison's argument, he might respond like this:

"I understand that you're advocating for a greater investment in renewable energy because of the significant environmental costs associated with fossil fuels, which include air pollution and the contribution to climate change. It's true that solar and wind power offer cleaner alternatives that could reduce our carbon footprint and reliance on nonrenewable resources. Let's explore how we can increase our renewable energy capacity while also ensuring that we have reliable energy available at all times, even when the sun isn't shining or the wind isn't blowing. Could we discuss the role of energy storage technologies and grid improvements in achieving this balance?"

Steelmanning fosters a more nuanced and productive dialogue, focusing on addressing potential challenges and finding effective solutions.

THE BODY (POLITIC) IN BALANCE

Social Homeostasis

Like the human body thrives in the Goldilocks zone, so does the body politic. Biological homeostasis is the ability of an organism to regulate its internal environment to maintain a stable, constant condition, despite external fluctuations.

Social homeostasis refers to the processes and mechanisms through which societies maintain stability, balance, and cohesion in the face of internal and external changes or stresses.

In a social context, homeostasis involves various regulatory processes that help a society manage and adapt to challenges such as economic fluctuations, political upheaval, environmental changes, or social tensions. The aim is to preserve the social structure, ensure the well-being of its members, and maintain the group's overall functionality and harmony.

This is not a political tome, but you don't have to hold a Ph.D. in sociology to be acutely aware of the current political invective. Both "sides" have slid to the thinner edges of the branch. Our society looks much like a frayed shoelace, bulging at the far extremes and holding on tenuously by a thread in the center. We know that health, in all its expressions, is a reflection of balance, of a strong and resilient middle. This is why having difficult, compassionate conversations is so important.

As I underscored in Part I, we live in mutual interdependence. We cannot separate the behavior of an organism from the behavior of its environment. Our physiology both influences and is influenced by its ecosystem. Similarly, we cannot separate our psycho-social selves from the greater social fabric. We are sculpted by our environment while also shaping it. Such is always the relationship between the part and the whole.

CHAPTER 17

SHELTERED IN PLACE

Loneliness & Social Fitness

Loneliness is the ultimate poverty.

— Pauline Esther Phillips

It was a nightly ritual for Ffej and his tribe to gather around a crackling fire as the sun dipped and the air cooled. On most days, resources could be gathered across four to six hours, which left time to gather, eat, and share stories of the day. Communal life provided camaraderie, but it was also essential for survival.

Some members of the group kept watch at night to protect fellow tribesmen from predators. Other members hunted and foraged for game, plants, fruits, roots, tubers, and seeds for the clan. Tribes moved around together as resources in one area became picked over. This led to collective "family planning" as tribe size needed to be kept small and stable. Mothers breastfed their babies for extended periods of time for myriad reasons. Breast milk served as "free" food, and under ancestral conditions of hunting, gathering, and high infant mortality, infant survival depended on the immunological, hormonal, and nutritional factors found in maternal breast milk. Prolonged breastfeeding also served as a means of natural contraception as the practice decreased female fertility. This contributed to a stable population over tens of thousands of years.

Communal child-rearing was commonplace. The babies of *Homo sapiens* are unique in their sustained and unqualified reliance on their caretakers. Compare this dependence with other animals. Most normal foals, for example, will stand within 40 minutes to 1 hour of being born.[1] Baby robins jump from their nest when they are about 13 days old. It takes them another 10 or so days to become strong fliers and independent birds.[2] At six weeks of age, a human baby can only see about 12 inches away. And it will be another year before it gets up on its legs and walks.[3] And not that skillfully. This phenomenon may be due to an evolutionary tension.

Evolution & Community

While the timeline is not particularly clear, it appears that *Australopithecus*, an early hominin, took their first steps as committed bipeds between 2 and 4 million years ago.[4] Bipedalism resulted in skeletal changes to the legs, knee and ankle joints, spine, toes, and arms. Most significantly, the hips tapered and the pelvis became shorter and rounded. In female hominins, this led to a narrower birth canal.

The chronology of the human mastery of fire is equally mangy. The oldest unequivocal evidence, found at Israel's Qesem cave, dates back 300,000 to 400,000 years.[5] The ability to control fire altered the course of human history in various ways, the most significant of which was cooking. Prior to cooking, it was not uncommon for hominins to spend a good part of the day chewing. Our primate ancestors give us a window into the time allocated for mastication. Chimps chew for 4.5 hours per day, and orangutans clock 6.6 hours. Modern humans spend a mere 35 minutes every day chewing.[6] Uncooked food needs a tremendous amount of breaking down and predigestion. Further, the metabolism of raw food requires a tremendous amount of energy.

Cooking changed the equation. The chemical transformations induced through cooking made it easier for our bodies to digest carbohydrates, proteins, and fats. It reduced the need for incessant chewing and expanded nature's pantry to include foods that were previously inedible or very difficult to digest, including grains, tubers, maize, and meats.

With the advent of cooking, hominins unearthed a surfeit of excess calories.[7] This discovery went to our heads, quite literally.

The average brain size of *Australopithecus* was 400 cubic centimeters. Between 1 and 2 million years ago, the brain size of *Homo erectus* doubled. Currently, *Homo sapiens* boast brains of approximately 1,300 cubic centimeters. When it comes to energy, our brains are greedy devils, pilfering 20 percent of our available ATP, even though they have only 2 percent of our body mass.[8]

You might presage where these two convergent evolutionary trends were headed. Bigger brains and narrower birth canals led to increasingly difficult and perilous childbirth. It is theorized that this resulted in shorter gestation periods as babies needed to be born before their heads became too large. In comparison to other animals, one could argue that human babies are born premature. Certainly, they are helpless. Given their utter reliance on others and the conditions of hunter-gatherer life, babies required multiple caregivers.

The phrase "it takes a village to raise a child" originates from an African proverb and conveys the message that it requires a community to provide a safe, healthy environment for children to develop and flourish.

Evolutionary pressure led to collective child-rearing. By dint of our biology, we are obliged to support each other. Ffej and his fellow tribespeople couldn't survive in single-family households. Of course, communal living is the manner in which we existed for the overwhelming majority of human history. We lived in large camps, depending on one another for food, childcare, and virtually everything else—all without walls, doors, or picket fences.

One day recently in Topanga, Gabor Maté said to me, "If the entirety of human history was reduced to one day, we lived communally for 23 hours and 54 minutes of it."

Community is an adaptive advantage. Humans are not the fastest or most muscular creatures on Earth. What makes humans unique, and shot us to the top of the food chain, is our ability to cooperate flexibly at scale.

Modernity has mischaracterized the notion of "survival of the fittest." The phrase has come to connote a world of cutthroat competition in which only strong individuals will succeed and the weak will perish. But survival doesn't favor individualism. Our ability to survive and thrive is bound to our capacity to function collectively.

The fittest—and happiest—of us are those who can foster deep social connection.

When we say things like, "it's just human nature to be selfish and egocentric and look out for one's needs first," we confuse nature with culture. Yes, it's our culture to be individualistic, but our nature is communal. And when we defy nature, it rarely works to our advantage.

The last 300 years in the West have been dominated by the sanctification of the individual. Yuval Harari chronicles this trend masterfully in his book *Sapiens*. Romanticism implores the individual to follow one's heart and satisfy their wanderlust. Art bequeaths beauty to the eye of the beholder. Commerce yields to the customer who is always right. Liberal democracy gives every citizen a vote—most of the time. Even physics points to the individual subjectivity of experience.

Our modern heroes are the rugged individuals, the Marlboro men, the captains of industry, the star athletes, the winners of social Darwinism. But individualism comes with a cost.

We live increasingly alone—atomized, living in boxes within boxes within boxes. Our children barricade themselves in their rooms within picket-fenced houses cloistered in gated communities.

The initial boom of single-family homes took place in the early 20th century, facilitated by new building technologies and materials. After World War II, the middle class became increasingly enchanted by the lure of suburbia. Developments like Levittown in New York, where mass-produced homes were built on a large scale, marked a significant moment in the history of single-family residential housing. Detached homes with yards, garages, and multiple bedrooms and bathrooms became a symbol of social status and personal success.

According to the Roots of Loneliness Project, 52 percent of Americans report feeling lonely while 47 percent report their relationships with others are not meaningful. And 58 percent of Americans reported that they sometimes or always feel like no one knows them well. Astoundingly, single or not, 57 percent of Americans report eating all meals alone.[9] Fewer than three people live in the average American household.[10]

What are the physiological and psychological impacts of loneliness?

People are generally aware of the most common health indicators and risk factors. We don't always heed our own advice, but we understand that poor diet, smoking, alcohol use, sedentariness, and obesity pose risks. What we might not know is that social isolation is just as predictive of death.

BYU professors Tim Smith and Julianne Holt-Lunstad have conducted research that demonstrates that loneliness poses the same risk of death as smoking 15 cigarettes a day or being an alcoholic.[11] Their more recent study also reveals that the risk of social isolation surpasses that posed by obesity.[12]

Unfortunately, more people live alone today than at any time in human history. These data inspired Surgeon General Vivek Murthy, the country's top doctor, to declare loneliness an epidemic and author a book on the topic.

Loneliness directly interacts with the wiring of our nervous system. Being lonely induces a stress state through increasing the human perception of threat. Our brain innately knows that there is greater security in groups. We grok this reality as a product of direct experience. Imagine the feeling of getting lost in the wilderness by yourself versus losing your way with a group. Your limbic system innately understands that your chances of survival are greater in a group. Modern society can feel like a wilderness for many people.

The downstream impacts of loneliness-induced stress include chronic fatigue, brain fog, high glucose levels, gut dysbiosis, systemic inflammation, diabetes, and cardiovascular disease. The persistent activation of the sympathetic nervous system creates hormonal imbalances in the body that can lead to these conditions and others. The overactivation of steroid hormones produced in the adrenal glands such as cortisol and adrenaline can spike glucose levels, lower immune function, and disrupt the balance of gut flora.

Social isolation can even impact gene expression. Sociogenomics is an emerging field that studies epigenetics in relation to the social environment. In other words, our gene expression is in some measure dependent on social interaction. Individuals who suffer from chronic loneliness have different transcriptome profiles for genes related to immune system factors, including elevated expression of pro-inflammatory cytokine genes and decreased expression of antiviral genes. Chronically isolated individuals are also more likely to develop inflammation-related diseases, thus providing a plausible biological connection between social variables and disease risk and mortality.

When threat perception increases, we begin to question people's motives. Trust erodes, and our focus shifts inward. Under perceived threat, humans develop an excessive focus on self. In this sense, loneliness has contributed to erosion of social trust that is tearing at the fabric of our society.

Loneliness is also a downward spiral. The lonelier we are, the more we believe that we are unworthy and unlikeable. As our self-esteem plummets, we are more likely to seek out self-destructive external agents to assuage our perceived deficiencies, find relief, and create a sense of connection. Turning to the comfort of alcohol or drugs becomes a way of coping with feeling alone, unloved, and rejected. Substance use is an anesthetic for pain. But, of course, they provide only short-term reprieve.

Substance abuse helps to avoid confronting problems, delivering a false, brief sense of security. It is a vicious cycle because when the drugs and alcohol are not present, all our emotions come flooding back in.

Loneliness and addiction are bidirectional, fueling each other in equal and horrifying measure. As addiction worsens, many people damage relationships and lose friends, further aggravating loneliness and isolation. In the absence of support, it is incredibly difficult to cope with those feelings without drugs or alcohol—so the cycle continues. In this sense, loneliness is both an effect and a cause of addiction.

Of course, we are aware of the psychological impacts of social isolation. Isolation is leveraged by our justice system. The most severe punishment doled out short of a death sentence is solitary confinement.

We are still getting our collective heads around the long-term effects of the forced monasticism imposed by the COVID pandemic. We've seen a dreadful increase in suicide rates and drug overdoses.

That said, rates of loneliness were skyrocketing prior to COVID putting its wicked foot on the accelerator.

In the absence of in-real-life interaction, we have resorted to creating "connection" from behind screens. However, study after study suggests that social media actually exacerbates feelings of isolation instead of fostering social bonds.

Online interactions lack the nonverbal cues, physical presence, and emotional intimacy that are essential for building and maintaining meaningful relationships. Social media can also lead to feelings of comparison and inadequacy as well as feelings of isolation due to constant FOMO (fear of missing out).

Loneliness can be both objective and subjective. Objective loneliness is a reflection of social isolation and having very few, if any, social connections. Subjective loneliness stems from a feeling that the social bonds you do have fall short of your social needs. We can be around people and still feel lonely. We've likely all had the feeling at one time or another of being lonely in a crowd or at a party.

The Reverend Michael Beckwith once told me in an interview, "Loneliness is often a loneliness with yourself."

We've probably all been in conversations where the person with whom we're speaking is looking over our shoulder, scanning the room for someone more "important" to ensnare. This tendency is a reflection of lack of self-worth. The incessant seeking out of the approval of others inhibits the ability for people to be present and connect. This is a form of loneliness with oneself.

It's important to delineate between loneliness and solitude. The latter is a form of chosen aloneness that can be the source of replenishment and feel extremely connective. In fact, meditation can elicit a sensation of oneness and interpenetration with the world. In a deep meditative state, the separation between the external world and your internal reality dissipates. The sense that you are sitting somewhere on the edge of experience, looking in at it, dissolves. This transcendent feeling is also the product of immersion into nature or creative expression.

It is ironic that the pathway to developing greater connection to the external world is often forged in periods of solitude. Ultimately, we seek a reality in which we complete ourselves and don't feel lonely when we're alone. And, at the same time, we bring our confident and authentic selves into the world around us.

Robert Waldinger is a professor of psychiatry at Harvard Medical School and the director of the Harvard Study of Adult Development, the world's longest and most comprehensive study of human happiness. Launched in 1938, the longitudinal study followed 238 college sophomores (and their progeny) across 85 years. When I asked Robert for the number one determinant of self-reported happiness and well-being, he responded without hesitation, "Hands-down, the strength of one's social connections."

While Ffej enjoyed his moments of solitude and introspection, he had very little occasion to be lonely. He felt a profound sense of accountability to the tribe and, in return, possessed a deep sense of belonging, of being accepted as his authentic self.

Just like Ffej didn't need to work out to remain strong and flexible, Ffej's social fitness was a product of his lifestyle.

Loneliness is like thirstiness. It's a signal. It's a reflection that your social connections are not meeting your social needs. Too many of us have no one to confide in, to call in an emergency or with whom to vulnerably talk through problems.

Our modern culture is peppered with the trapdoors of loneliness. We need to treat social fitness like cardiovascular fitness and actively engage in the activities that foster greater connection and mimic the circumstances in which we evolved.

The Protocols of Social Fitness

One hundred pull-ups. One hundred push-ups. One hundred sit-ups. These are my daily fitness nonnegotiables. Of course, I'll work in some tennis when scheduling allows. Chasing yellow fuzzy balls like a golden retriever might be considered play, but fortunately it is also fantastic for cardiovascular health.

Many of us have fitness regimes. We commit to the gym, the track, or the court to keep our bodies strong and flexible.

But what about the atrophy of our social muscles? I've described modernity's scourge of loneliness. Given that social isolation is as detrimental to health as alcohol or smoking 15 cigarettes per day, many of us must now impose a social fitness regimen to accompany our biceps curls.

As a means to improve social connectivity, I have assembled a social fitness regimen. Many of these practices may seem very simple, however, the net impact is inestimable.

Five minutes every day: In 1987, AT&T released a commercial set to the jingle, "Reach out and touch someone." Billy has gone off to college and is feeling lonely and nostalgic. He pecks out his home number on the analog keypad and his mother picks up. Billy is lighthearted, but his mother senses his wistfulness. Billy feels heard and seen.

Take five minutes every day to connect with a relative or friend. Like the vegetables in your garden, your relationships cannot thrive unless they are nurtured. If needed, you can set an automatic reminder on your incredibly smart phone.

Answer the phone: Pick up when a loved one rings even if you "can't talk." Instead of exchanging an endless stream of texts, tell them that you'll return their call as soon as possible.

Forge in-person connection: Don't mistake virtual connection for the real thing. Despite the ever-increasing opportunities to connect online, Americans report having fewer friends than they did decades ago. Connection relies on more than the content of what someone is saying. We evolved to "dance" in conversation. We read body language and vocal intonation. We connect through eye contact, mimicking body movements, nodding along, and, of course, through offering each other touch and physical affection.

Practice Random Acts of Kindness: These acts are spontaneous and unpremeditated gestures of friendliness and generosity. They are often simple. A smile to a stranger, public recognition of a co-worker, picking up litter on the street, or leaving a good tip. These deeds may seem small and token, but what is the human condition except an aggregate of billions of small actions?

Cultivate compassion: Identify someone else's suffering as your own and actively work to alleviate that pain. Compassion is an experience of interbeing. When you viscerally feel someone else's pain, you transcend self and feel connected to something bigger.

Empathetic joy: Experience joy solely for someone else's joy without envy or jealousy. When we witness the achievements of others, we often project our feelings of our own unfulfilled potential onto that person. This results in envy or resentment. Don't compare. Celebrate the accomplishments of others.

Serve: Service to others through volunteering or providing assistance plays a crucial role in social fitness. Serving others can increase empathy and understanding as it often involves interacting with individuals who may be different from us or in situations unlike our own. We can find deep satisfaction in knowing that we are making a positive difference in the lives of others. Service activities often involve collaborating with others, which can create opportunities for social connection. This can help individuals feel more connected to their communities and can foster a sense of social belonging.

Build communication skills: In my 20s, I ran a record label, and our music was big in Japan. I traveled to Tokyo many times for business. My trips were packed with meetings with record executives. I would ramble on and on, passionately extolling the virtues of a new record or signing. When I finished, there was nothing. Silence. Of course, at first, the lack of response was discombobulating, and I felt the need to awkwardly fill the emptiness. Eventually, I learned that the pregnant pause was actually an indication of respect. My counterpart had listened thoroughly and was now processing an appropriate response.

The Japanese listen to understand, not to respond. When someone else is talking, we tend to formulate our rejoinder and only partially listen. Try to pay full attention to others without any compulsion to reply. Show others that you are invested in their feelings through active listening.

At the same time, when you do speak, practice clear, assertive, and respectful communication. This includes both verbal and nonverbal cues, such as body language and tone of voice.

Foster conflict resolution skills: You can practice the middle way by bringing opposing positions together. Reframe the concept of "winning" away from trying to elicit an admission of defeat and toward fostering compromise and cooperation. Admit when you're wrong and say you're sorry. Learn to forgive and move on.

Give the gift of presence: In the age of the attention economy in which everyone and everything is vying for your conscious attention, the most precious gift you can give anyone is the present of presence. Be all there.

Teach through example: While our children and loved ones may never listen to us, they rarely fail to imitate us. Oftentimes, we want our influence to be explicit and direct but never underestimate the immeasurable value of just being there every day, of leading a life of example, of walking an honorable, if occasionally jagged, path such that there are footsteps in which to follow.

Solitude: Ironically, deliberate solitude is a means to social fitness. The French philosopher Blaise Pascal wrote, "All of humanity's problems stem from man's inability to sit quietly in a room alone." So many of us are simply not comfortable alone. We immediately fidget or grab our phone. However, connection to self is a bridge to social connection.

The Golden Rule is a spiritual axiom shared among myriad traditions. It instructs us to "love thy neighbor as thyself." Yes, this maxim asks us to be charitable and altruistic. However, in order to fulfill this timeless equation, we must also love ourselves. We must belong to ourselves, accepting ourselves for who we are. This is no easy feat but it begins with being comfortable in our aloneness. Eventually, in fulfilling our own needs, in becoming complete, love can become something given, not taken.

Let me punctuate the "stressful" practice of chosen solitude with this magnificent quote from Rainer Maria Rilke's, *Letters to a Young Poet*:[13]

> And you should not let yourself be confused in your solitude by the fact that there is something in you that wants to move out of it. This very wish, if you use it calmly and prudently and like a tool, will help you spread out your solitude over a great distance. Most people have (with the help

of conventions) turned their solutions toward what is easy and toward the easiest side of the easy; but it is clear that we must trust in what is difficult; everything alive trusts in it, everything in Nature grows and defends itself any way it can and is spontaneously itself, tries to be itself at all costs and against all opposition. We know little, but that we must trust in what is difficult is a certainty that will never abandon us; it is good to be solitary, for solitude is difficult; that something is difficult must be one more reason for us to do it.

THE BODY IN BALANCE

Becoming an Ambivert

Social fitness is a delicate balance between extraversion and introversion. Most of us feel a tendency toward one or the other. Some of us are more outgoing, socially confident, and gain energy from being around people, while others are generally quiet, introspective, and generate energy from spending time alone.

Extraverts are often comfortable in group settings and enjoy engaging in social activities. They're typically more assertive, expressive, and tend to enjoy seeking out new experiences. Introverts often prefer one-on-one conversations or solitary activities to large social gatherings. They typically spend more time thinking and reflecting and are more reserved in expressing their feelings or thoughts.

The most socially fit are ambiverts. They balance a desire and ability to bond with others while fostering the powers of introspection and finding connection in solitude.

Social connection is inextricably linked to psychological and physiological well-being. Make social fitness a priority.

CHAPTER 18

EATING STRESSED PLANTS

Xenohormetins

What doesn't kill plants may make us stronger.

— MICHAEL GREGER, M.D.

In the fall of 2022, Dr. Jeffrey Bland paid Commune Topanga a visit. Jeff is like the "Lucy" of functional medicine. Virtually every doctor I have interviewed traces their epistemological ancestry back to Jeffrey Bland, who worked directly with Linus Pauling and brought the field of functional medicine to the fore in 1991. His influence on modern medical science is inestimable.

As we sat jawing on the patio, Jeffrey reached into a canvas tote and pulled out two taut five-pound paper bags. He plopped them down on the table, producing a small cloud of particulate matter.

He pointed to the bags, his transcendent blue eyes becoming starry, and declared, "This is the most stressed plant in the world."

The stress of frigid temperatures, scorching sun, blistering wind, drought, and other inhospitable environmental conditions evidently don't exclusively apply to humans and other animals. Plants, too, can get stressed. As we've seen, in response to short-term stress, humans have evolved adaptive mechanisms that result in greater resiliency. Hormesis is the biological phenomenon where a beneficial effect—such as improved health, stress tolerance, growth, or longevity—results from exposure to low doses of an agent that is otherwise toxic or lethal when given at higher doses.

It turns out that plants also have a hormetic response to stress. In response to hostile growing conditions, plants generate protective compounds known as xenohormetins. These phytochemicals are also referred to as polyphenols. The protective qualities of xenohormetins are then transferred to humans when we consume them. These compounds have been associated with anti-inflammatory, antioxidant, and anticancer effects.

By contrast, conventional agriculture with its chemical fertilizers, heavy irrigation, pesticides, and herbicides produce brittle and nutrient-deficient plants. Industrial agriculture is to plants what McDonald's is to people. Yes, it's convenient for a plant to grow in the absence of weeds and pests, with abundant water and neatly organized rank on rank. But a dearth of struggle will turn a russet potato into a . . . couch potato.

Dr. Jeffrey Bland claims to have found the world's most stressed plant. It's called Himalayan tartary buckwheat (HTB). It evolved unsurprisingly in the Himalayas, a notoriously inhospitable place for plants. For millennia, this gluten-free food crop, which has no relation to wheat, has weathered harsh climes, high altitudes, and poor-quality soil. Yet HTB has become more robust—physically and genetically—as a direct result of these suboptimal conditions. And when we eat HTB, we unlock a treasure trove of unique nutrients, including antioxidant polyphenols like quercetin, rutin, and luteolin that help contribute to an effective immune response. HTB also contains 2-HOBA, a rare plant nutrient that has been found to protect the human body's proteins from harmful biological aging processes.

Examples of other xenohormetins include resveratrol from red wine, curcumin from turmeric, and sulforaphane from cruciferous vegetables. Resveratrol, for example, developed naturally in grape skins to fight fungus. Many winemakers deliberately stress their grapes, often growing them in arid conditions. They do this not for phytochemical purposes but for taste.

Resveratrol when ingested by humans activates SIRT1, one of the proteins in the sirtuin family. Sirtuins influence a wide range of cellular processes like aging, transcription, apoptosis, inflammation, stress resistance, energy efficiency during low-calorie situations, and mitochondrial biogenesis.

Curiously, the most stressed grape is the pinot noir varietal. By extension, you will find the greatest concentration of resveratrol in a glass of pinot. But don't pop the cork just yet. You'd need to drink 1,000 bottles of wine a day to fulfill the recommended dosage of resveratrol. This is not recommended.

Sirtuins are unique because they require a coenzyme called nicotinamide adenine dinucleotide (NAD) to function. NAD levels decline as we age, and this decline is thought to be one of the contributing factors to aging and age-associated diseases. This is why it is increasingly popular to supplement with NAD or its precursor nicotinamide mononucleotide (NMN).

Much of the research on sirtuins has been done by the Australian biologist Dr. David Sinclair. Sinclair is a professor in the department of genetics at Harvard Medical School and co-director of the Paul F. Glenn Center for the Biology of Aging. He is best known for his research on aging and longevity, particularly in relation to activating the sirtuin pathway in yeast. Whether resveratrol has the same impact on human longevity as it does on yeast remains a very open question.

Another overly anxious plant is green tea. Japanese matcha is a type of powdered green tea, grown in a traditional way. Growing the plants in the shade stresses them, causing them to make biologically active compounds, including theanine, caffeine, chlorophyll, and various types of catechins, including epigallocatechin gallate (ECGC) that boost the activity of defense enzymes such as SIRT1. Sipping matcha green tea helps burn fat, protects the kidneys, improves memory, decreases inflammation, and is anti-carcinogenic.

Stressed plants abound in the blue zone. The blue zone, originally identified by author Dan Buettner, are the five places in the world with the greatest prevalence of centenarians. They are Okinawa, Japan; Sardinia, Italy; Nicoya, Costa Rica; Ikaria, Greece; and Loma Linda, California.[1] These longevity hubs all share certain characteristics, including limited technology, healthy diets, active outdoor cultures, community, hilliness, and—yes—stressed plants. The living conditions of the blue zone are modernity's best proxy of how Ffej lived some 12,000 years ago. Not only do the denizens of the blue zone eat a plethora of nutrient-dense plants, but the animals that they eat graze on these plants as well.

You may notice that two of the world's blue zone are islands in the Mediterranean Sea. The famed Mediterranean diet has been associated with longevity. Extra-virgin olive oil (EVOO) is a staple of the regimen. There is a bioactive compound in olive oil called oleocanthal. Oleocanthal has potent anti-inflammatory and antioxidant properties and may inhibit cancer-promoting genes.

As discussed in an earlier chapter, aging is highly associated with an imbalance between the AMPK and mTOR. This disequilibrium is driven by the overactivation of mTOR and by a decline in responsiveness to the activation of the energy-sensing protein AMPK, the body's clean up and repair pathway. Extra-virgin olive oil has been shown to activate AMPK.

The term *superfood* isn't always helpful as it can lead people to overconsume one specific food at the expense of eating the rainbow. I personally attempt to eat 30 different types of vegetables per week. Still, there is a good case to be made for olive oil as a member of the food pantheon.

Protocollards

Sprouting Inconvenience

If you really want to inconvenience yourself into better health, then allow me to unveil the world's most nutrient-dense food: sprouts.

I was introduced to the wondrous world of sprouting by the self-appointed "sprout king," Doug Evans, whose irrepressible zeal for the practice is matched only by a retriever's zest for chasing soggy tennis balls.

When I first met Doug, he bounded toward me. He opened his hand to reveal a solitary broccoli seed, brown and oval shaped with a conspicuous white spot on one flank. It appeared almost microscopic in the middle of his palm, no more than 1 millimeter in diameter. Given the right conditions, however, this wee seed would grow into a 7-inch wide broccoli head composed of distinct florets. But he had other plans for it. And has now inculcated me into the sprouting cult.

One can sprout seeds of myriad species, including but not limited to alfalfa, clover, fenugreek, turnip green, wheat grass, wild rice, green pea, radish, adzuki beans, lentil, chickpeas, mung beans, and red cabbage, among others.

The equipment requirements for sprouting are negligible: a wide-mouthed quart-sized mason jar, some cheesecloth, and a rubber band. Sure, you can purchase kits that incorporate metal holsters that secure the mason jars at a 45-degree angle to facilitate proper drainage, but it's hardly necessary. You can stack your sprouting jars on a dish drying rack, among other improvisations.

Two tablespoons of these miniscule broccoli seeds will yield a pound of sprouts in four to six days. The labor is hardly onerous. You soak the seeds for six to eight hours, put the jars in a cool and shady spot, and then simply rinse and drain them twice per day. It's immensely gratifying to watch the seeds push forth their tiny white stems and green dollhouse-sized leaves.

This process of germination is pre-photosynthetic. The seedling is leveraging warehoused energy, a small parcel of food stored in the endosperm of the seed. These stockpiled nutrients—starch, fats and proteins—can lay dormant within the seed for thousands of years. But given the right conditions—moisture, air, and a moderate temperature—the embryo will be activated to grow, cracking through the dampened seed coat and . . . sprout.

Sprouts, specifically broccoli sprouts, are considered the most nutrient-dense food in the world. The concentration of phytochemicals in broccoli sprouts is 40 times that of broccoli florets.[2] They are also low calorie, organic, and fiber-rich. What's more is that they also may be Earth's most anti-carcinogenic food due to the compound sulforaphane.

Xenohormetins, which confer benefits when consumed, co-evolved in relation to their environment. Good stress—sun, wind, rocky soils, and weeds in the right dosage—built resilience. And what is true for plants turns out to be remarkably true for humans.

Eat the Rainbow of Stress

Here's my list of some well-known xenohormetins, their benefits, and their "stressed" hosts:

Resveratrol

Source: Grapes (especially in the skins), red wine, peanuts, and berries
Benefits: Linked to anti-aging effects, cardiovascular health, and neuroprotective properties

Sulforaphane

Source: Cruciferous vegetables like broccoli, Brussels sprouts, cabbages, and broccoli sprouts
Benefits: Antioxidant and detoxification properties, potential anticancer effects

Curcumin

Source: Turmeric root
Benefits: Anti-inflammatory, antioxidant, and potential neuroprotective effects

Quercetin

Source: Onions, apples, grapes, berries, tea and, Himalayan tartary buckwheat
Benefits: Antioxidant, anti-inflammatory, and potential cardiovascular benefits

Epigallocatechin Gallate (EGCG)

Source: Green tea
Benefits: Antioxidant properties, linked to weight management and cardiovascular health

Piceatannol

Source: Grapes, berries, and passion fruit
Benefits: Similar to resveratrol, with potential anti-inflammatory and anticancer activities

Salidroside

Source: Rhodiola rosea (an herb in the Rhodiola genera)
Benefits: Adaptogenic effects, enhancing stress resistance, anti-fatigue, and potential neuroprotective properties

Oleuropein

Source: Olive leaves and olives
Benefits: Cardiovascular benefits, antioxidant, and anti-inflammatory properties

Fisetin

Source: Strawberries, apples, and persimmons
Benefits: Antioxidant, neuroprotective, and potential anti-aging effects

Kaempferol

Source: Tea, broccoli, kale, and beans
Benefits: Antioxidant and potential anticancer properties

Luteolin

Source: Peppers, carrots, celery, olive oil, and Himalayan tartary buckwheat
Benefits: Anti-inflammatory, antioxidant, and neuroprotective effects

THE BODY IN BALANCE

Antioxidants & Free Radicals

As described, in response to harsh environmental circumstances such as wind, cold, scorching sun, and compromised soil, plants generate protective mechanisms to ensure survival. These xenohormetic plants develop certain antioxidant compounds that we call polyphenols that shield them from threat. These protective attributes are then transferred to humans when we eat them.

Antioxidants and free radicals are two opposing forces in the body that play a significant role in maintaining health and preventing disease.

A free radical is one of the more entertaining terms in biology. It conjures images of long-locked, tie-dyed hippies advocating for social change while gnawing on grilled cheese. Indeed, a free radical is a molecule who yearns to shake up the system. Just like Moonbeam's birth name was more than likely something akin to Judith Goldstein, free radicals are in some cases known by their more formal designation as reactive oxygen species (ROS). A free radical is a molecule capable of independent existence that contains an unpaired electron in its atomic orbital. This results in instability and hyper-reactivity. It's so tempting to keep the hippie metaphor going here, but I'll resist. In any case, they can either donate an electron to or accept an electron from other molecules, therefore behaving as oxidants or reductants.

The most important oxygen-containing free radicals in many disease states are hydroxyl radical, superoxide anion radical, hydrogen peroxide, oxygen singlet, hypochlorite, nitric oxide radical, and peroxynitrite radical. These are highly reactive molecules capable of wreaking havoc on other cells, including damaging DNA.

Free radicals are derived from normal metabolic processes in the human body. Just being alive and making ATP produces a certain quantity of them. Free radicals are also generated in response to external agents such as exposure to X-rays, ozone, cigarette smoking, air pollutants, and industrial chemicals.

If reactive oxygen species are the free-wheeling hippies of the body, then antioxidants are their straitlaced suburban cousins. An antioxidant is a molecule stable enough to donate an electron to a rampaging free radical and neutralize it, thus reducing its capacity to do damage. Antioxidants delay or inhibit cellular damage mainly through this free radical scavenging function.

Oxidative Stress

The term *oxidative stress* is used to describe the condition of oxidative damage resulting when the critical balance between free radical generation and antioxidant defenses is unfavorable. This disequilibrium arises as a result of an imbalance between free radical and antioxidant production.

Oxidative stress is involved with a wide host of physiological and neurological disorders, including cancer, heart disease, Parkinson's, autism, depression, and others.[3] In the case of cancer, for example, free radicals can induce DNA damage, which can lead to the production and proliferation of dysfunctional cells. Antioxidants can decrease oxidative stress–induced carcinogenesis through the aforementioned process of scavenging reactive oxygen species.[4]

The body endogenously produces some (enzymatic and non-enzymatic) antioxidants like glutathione, melatonin, uric acid, and superoxide dismutase. Other antioxidants must be consumed through diet, primarily through eating plants.

While glutathione receives most of the headlines as your body's chief endogenously produced antioxidant, melatonin may be just as potent despite its second billing. Melatonin is famously known as the sleep hormone and is secreted into the bloodstream by the pineal gland. At the mitochondrial level, however, it is also a powerful antioxidant and protects the crucial organelle from free radical damage. Humans can upregulate the production of mitochondrial melatonin through light exposure, specifically to near-infrared spectrum light as described in the chapter about light therapy.

Plant-Derived Antioxidants

In the 19th century, British sailors earned the nickname "limeys" among American naval cadets. This derogatory epithet was due to lime and lemon juice rations doled out by the Royal Navy to ward off scurvy.[5] American sailors hadn't yet discovered the administration of vitamin C as a preventative treatment. Arrr . . . the scurvy.

Vitamin C, a.k.a. ascorbic acid, has utility beyond protecting sailors from the ravages of life at sea. Humans, unlike most animals, are unable to synthesize vitamin C endogenously, so it is an essential dietary component. Vitamin C is required for the biosynthesis of collagen, L-carnitine, and certain neurotransmitters. It is also involved in protein metabolism. But it is a powerful, if unheralded, antioxidant found in the aforementioned citrus fruits, tomatoes, potatoes, red and green peppers, kiwifruit, broccoli, strawberries, Brussels sprouts, and cantaloupe.

Citrus fruits are also a significant source of flavanols, like quercetin, as are apples, onions, parsley, sage, tea, red wine, olive oil, grapes, dark cherries, and dark berries such as blueberries and blackberries.

Vegetables and fruits such as celery, parsley, broccoli, onion leaves, carrots, peppers, cabbages, apple skins, and chrysanthemum flowers are rich in luteolin. And high concentrations of catechins can be found in coffee, tea, red wine, broad beans, black grapes, apricots, and strawberries.

Drinking Coke & Free Radical Production

If plants provide health-conferring properties to humans through antioxidants, then they are in a tug-of-war with excessive glucose consumption.

A recent study published by a number of endocrinologists at the University of Buffalo demonstrated that glucose intake increases production of free radicals and lowers levels of antioxidants.[6] In the study, 75 grams of glucose, the simplest form of sugar, was dissolved in 300 milliliters of water and given to 14 healthy men and women. This is roughly the equivalent of glucose in two cans of Coke. Another six participants, who served as controls, drank a water-saccharin solution. Results showed there was no change in free-radical generation in samples taken from controls. However, in samples from subjects who drank the sugar water, free radical generation increased significantly at one hour and more than doubled at two hours.

Jessie Inschaupe, a.k.a. the Glucose Goddess, also points articulately to this phenomenon in her books and on my podcast . . . as if we need another reason to reduce sugar consumption.

Like my crystal-laden hippie aunt, free radicals have their redeeming qualities. Reactive oxygen species are leveraged by the immune system to neutralize pathogens. And some short-term oxidative stress is hormetic. Like plants, humans develop protective mechanisms in response to just the right amount of stress. Again, disease and aging rear their heads in response to imbalances between free radicals and antioxidants. The key to health is fostering balance between these molecules through minimizing sugar consumption, eating vegetables, and exposure to the right light.

CHAPTER 19

REWILDING

Reconnecting with Nature

Though it can be easy to forget in our technologically advanced age, at our root, we're wild beings that, over time, have become domesticated.

— Tony Riddle

The National Three Peaks Challenge is a beast. It normally involves scaling the United Kingdom's three highest peaks, including the absurdly named Snowdon in Wales, Scafell Pike in England, and Ben Nevins in Scotland over a 24-hour period while driving 400 miles between the peaks.

Tony Riddle opted to put a little twist on it. In addition to climbing the peaks, he ran the entire distance between them in nine days, the equivalent of two marathons per day. And . . .

Tony did it all barefoot!

To make it more unfathomable, Tony Riddle was born with a clubfoot. At 44 years old, he became an ultra-endurance athlete and dedicated his life to seeking "freedom through natural movement." Tony is at the tip of the spear of a movement dubbed "human rewilding."

While the term *rewilding* is most commonly used in the context of ecological conservation, it can also apply to *Homo sapiens*. Human rewilding is the process of reconnecting people with nature and our own natural, ancestral behaviors. Nike inspired athletes to "Be like Mike." Rewilding's call-to-action is "Be like Ffej!"

The concept of rewilding is based on the belief that many modern lifestyle practices are mismatched with our evolutionary biology.

But fear not . . . human rewilding involves a variety of practices that happily don't require that you run 52.4 miles per day barefoot in the driving rain.

Rewilding can simply mean spending more time in the natural world. It would be difficult for the average Westerner to spend any less time immersed in nature. There are 1,440 minutes in the day. Currently the average Westerner spends 1,350 of them inside; 94 percent of our time is spent indoors or in a car.[1]

Forest Bathing

Shinrin-yoku, translated as "forest bathing," is a practice that came out of Japan in the 1980s. Forest bathing is not exercise, hiking, or jogging. It is simply connecting with nature through our senses of sight, hearing, taste, smell, and touch. By refining our instruments of perception, we bridge the gap between ourselves and the natural world and begin to sense ourselves as part of nature.

There is no strict regimented protocol for forest bathing. You simply find a park, trail, woods, or copse of trees. Lose your phone temporarily. Walk aimlessly and slowly as if your feet are kissing the ground. Listen intently to the polyphony of the myriad birds, the wind in the trees, and the rustling of animals in the underbrush. Inhale deeply through your nose. Notice the fragrances of flowers and wild grasses. Close your eyes halfway and witness the play of sunlight on the leaves. Caress the bark of trees. Dip your toes in a stream. Let nature in.

Forest bathing has been linked with multifarious health benefits. Spending time in nature lowers levels of cortisol, as well as blood pressure, heart rate, and muscle tension. Nature can help reduce feelings of anxiety, depression, and anger and boost mood and overall emotional well-being. Some research suggests that being in nature can increase levels of serotonin. Immersion in nature has been linked with improved attention, focus, and creativity. If you cannot access the great outdoors, even looking at pictures or videos of nature can improve focus and cognitive function.

When you're in nature, you're more likely to be physically active, which comes with a host of health benefits, including improved cardiovascular health, reduced risk of chronic diseases, and weight management. Research suggests that spending time in forest environments can enhance immune function, due to exposure to natural phytoncides (airborne chemicals produced by plants) that have antibacterial and antifungal qualities. Phytoncides may increase natural killer cells (NK cells), a type of leukocyte that supports the immune system and is linked with a lower risk of cancer. These white blood cells also fight infections and inflammation.

Spending time outside, especially in the morning, can help regulate your sleep-wake cycle, as described in detail in the chapter on light. Natural light exposure can help reset your circadian rhythm, leading to improved sleep quality. When your skin is exposed to sunlight, it manufactures vitamin D, which contributes to bone health, immune function, and mood regulation. Lastly, activities in nature often involve social interactions, which can improve feelings of social connectedness and contribute to mental well-being and feelings of gratitude.

You may have limited access to nature; 56 percent of the world's population now lives in a city.[2] Still, you can sensitize your awareness to the natural world. Recently, I came across a wee plant sprouting from an old tennis ball. By God, I thought, nature is irrepressible. I daydreamed of some future post-apocalyptic Earth in which a rainforest effloresced in an abandoned Macy's.

It's easy to become pessimistic and numb in the face of the enormity of the world's problems. But a blade of grass growing through the sidewalk's crack reminds us of the eternal reliability of nature. Nature is somewhere we can put our faith, not as belief in the absence of evidence but as trust in its inexorable quest to persist.

Lose the Shoes

Many hunter-gatherer societies likely went barefoot much of the time, especially in warmer climates. In harsher environments, some form of foot protection would have been necessary. For example, the Inuit and other Arctic aboriginal people wore mukluks, a soft boot traditionally made of reindeer skin or sealskin to protect them from frostbite. Others in rocky or thorny areas would have needed protection from cuts and punctures.

The oldest known footwear, a pair of sandals made from sagebrush fiber found in Oregon, is estimated to be around 10,000 years old. In general, though, while some hunter-gatherers developed footwear to adapt to different environments and weather conditions, most went shoeless.

A few years ago, I went hiking in the Santa Monica Mountains with Wim Hof, "the Iceman." In preparation, I laced up my cross-trainers nice and tight. But Wim did not. He embarked barefoot. Upon closer examination of his feet, I saw that they more resembled boots. They were tough, leathery, and broad. While stepping on a mere pebble might have caused me to squeal in pain, Wim's feet were inured to this type of insult. He happily ambled up the rocky trail without disturbance. Wim is a tree trunk of a man who appears impossible to knock over. This solidity is underwritten by the width of his feet that provide him with uncommon balance and steadiness.

The human foot is a biomechanical masterpiece. It contains 26 bones for natural stability; more than 100 muscles, tendons, and ligaments for strength and spring; and hundreds of thousands of nerve endings for sensory connection. Its complex structure of 33 joints is engineered both for weight-bearing and mobility. The architecture of the foot naturally allows for functions like standing, walking, running, and jumping.[3]

In modern society, we seldom go anywhere without binding our pedal masterworks in some form of leather, vinyl, or plastic. While shoes are important for protecting our feet in harsh environments or during intense physical activity, wearing shoes that are too tight, too narrow, too high, and too thick has numerous negative consequences.

Shoes do the work that muscles in the feet and lower legs would naturally do, which can lead to weaker foot and leg muscles over time. They reduce our natural range of motion. Shoes also reduce our ability to sense the ground beneath us, which is important for balance and body awareness. This sensory feedback is essential to preventing falls and injuries, which is particularly important as we age. According to the CDC, falls are the leading cause of injury-related death among adults age 65 and older. And the age-adjusted fall death rate increased by 41 percent from 55 per 100,000 older adults in 2012 to 78 per 100,000 older adults in 2021.[4]

Shoes alter our gait, often causing us to land on our heels, which is less natural and may increase the risk of injury. A midfoot strike allows your body to better absorb the force of impact, while running with a heel strike results in a more abrupt ground impact as the calf and Achilles are not able to absorb forces at ground contact.

Formal shoes, which have their origin in equestrianism, are dreadful for foot health. And, of course, women have it worse with high heels. These instruments of decorum cause bunions, hammertoes, corns, and calluses.

Most athletic shoes create a warm, dark, and moist environment, which is perfect for the growth of fungi. This dank milieu increases the risk of unsightly and malodorous conditions like athlete's foot and fungal nail infections.

Lastly, but not leastly, the production and disposal of shoes, particularly synthetic athletic shoes, has significant environmental impact. Every year in the United States, people discard 300 million pairs of shoes, 95 percent of which wind up in landfills, where they contaminate the environment by emitting chemicals, dyes, and adhesives into the soil and groundwater.[5]

According to my friend and eighth-generation cobbler, Galahad Clark, there are approximately 24 billion shoes bought annually around the world.

Remember Imelda Marcos's closet. She had 3,000 pairs of shoes—enough to wear a different pair every day for more than eight years! This takes foot fetishism to another level.

Going barefoot has pleiotropic benefits. Being barefoot improves your balance and posture as you are better able to sense the ground beneath you. Going barefoot can help strengthen the muscles in your feet and legs. This is because you're using more of the smaller muscles in your feet that are typically less engaged when you're wearing shoes.

Research suggests that going barefoot can reduce the risk of certain types of injuries, like ankle sprains or plantar fasciitis. It may also help alleviate some types of foot and knee pain. Many people find that going barefoot outside helps them feel more connected to nature and their environment. This can have psychological benefits, including stress reduction.

Stop Sitting Around & Squat

Before the efflorescence of desk jobs starting in the late 19th century, motor vehicles (invented in the 1890s), televisions (invented in 1927), and personal computers (invented in 1971), there was very little reason to sit. But, of course, these marvels of modernity are now ubiquitous and contribute to a glut of sedentary behavior. Other contributing factors include on-demand entertainment and the methods of learning promoted in our schools. Both of these phenomena have led to our children spending 10–12 hours per day staring at a glowing screen.[6]

The exact definition of a sedentary lifestyle is when someone spends six or more hours per day sitting or lying down. It is characterized by an energy expenditure ranging from 1 to 1.5 basal metabolic rate performed in a sitting or reclining posture.[7] Your basal metabolic rate is the number of calories you burn as your body performs the most basic life-sustaining functions.

One in four American adults sit for more than eight hours a day.[8] In England, adults of working age average about 9.5 hours per day of sedentary time. It increases with age. Between the ages of 65 and 74, sedentary time in both men and women increases to 10 hours per day or more. By age 75, people are sedentary for 11 hours per day.[9]

The lack of activity is, of course, a risk factor for health. Numerous studies have linked prolonged sitting with an increased risk of various chronic diseases, including heart disease, diabetes, and certain types of cancer. Sedentary behavior burns fewer calories compared to physical activity, which can contribute to weight gain and obesity. Research suggests that prolonged sitting can contribute to an increased risk of mental health issues, including depression and anxiety.

But it's not just about the dearth of physical exercise. Merely the act of sitting itself has negative implications.

Prolonged sitting, especially when done with poor posture, leads to back and neck pain and contributes to the development of musculoskeletal disorders. It weakens leg and gluteal muscles. It causes hip flexor muscles to shorten, leading to problems with hip joints. Long periods of sitting increases the risk of deep vein thrombosis, a condition where a blood clot forms in the lower legs.

To counteract the health risks associated with prolonged sitting, take regular breaks to stand up and walk. You can set your phone to remind you. Consider a standing or adjustable desk for work and aim to get regular exercise outside of work hours.

You can also eschew sitting altogether and opt for Ffej's default resting position: squatting. Of course, squatting is a very instinctive and natural position for both childbirth and pooping.

While Ffej was often moving from one task to another, hunter-gatherers did enjoy periods of inactivity. However, our ancestors' chillax time was often spent in postures like squatting that lead to higher levels of muscle activity than chair sitting.

Squatting for most modern humans is very difficult. Light Watkins, a wonderfully named meditation teacher, introduced me to the practice of squatting on one bright spring Topanga day. Light and I were deeply engaged in a conversation about the nature of consciousness. As I prattled on, I noticed that he remained in a resting squat position the entire time. Finally, I stopped blathering and asked him what he was doing. He encouraged me to try it.

I could barely hold a squat position for 20 seconds and couldn't get my heels remotely close to the ground. Light kindly wedged an available fire log under the soles of my feet for support.

"Start there," he exhorted, "and do it every day."

I have been squatting for a year now, and the benefits are incalculable. My hip flexors have opened up, my thighs are meaty and strong, and my balance is vastly improved.

Squatting increases ankle, hip, and spine mobility, leading to more stable and efficient movement. It involves the entire body, primarily targeting the quadriceps, hamstrings, and glutes but also engaging the core and lower back and, by extension, improving your posture.

Squatting requires and promotes flexibility in the lower back and hip complex, which can help prevent injuries and improve overall mobility. It requires a good deal of balance and coordination, which can carry over into improved performance in other sports and activities.

Like other weight-bearing exercises, squatting helps improve bone density, which is important for preventing osteoporosis. Squatting builds muscle. And the more muscle you have, the more calories your body burns at rest. This can help with weight management and metabolic health.

The moral of the story is this: Our divorce from nature is maladaptive. We seek out modern luxuries—be they temperature control or padded shoes or "easy" chairs. But, in the end, our creature comforts result in our physiological discomfiture. We are engineered for the Good Stress that nature provides.

Grounding

The word *grounding* carries assorted meanings—from dishing out punishment to obstreperous children to finding psychological equilibrium as one does when looking to ground oneself. Grounding is also a term relevant to electromagnetism. Electrical grounding is a fundamental safety feature in electrical systems. It involves creating a direct physical connection between electrical equipment and the earth. This connection is typically made using a conductor like copper or aluminum wire and is designed to protect both the equipment and the user from electrical faults.

Well, humans are, in a sense, a piece of electrical equipment too, as we produce a field of electrical charge. Further, emerging research suggests that there is potentially protective activity in "grounding" our bodies by directly connecting with the earth.[10]

Life coaches are constantly peddling positivity. Perhaps you've heard the axiom "change your thoughts, change your life." The belief is that affirmative thoughts will translate into beneficial behavior and also serve as a magnet for other positively minded people. This is commonly known as the law of attraction. While the notion that positivity attracts more positivity might work in psychology, it violates Coulomb's law of electromagnetism. The fundamental principle of this axiom is that like charges actually repel each other, while opposite charges attract one another.

In fact, a biologist might exhort you to "be more negative" as a means to reduce oxidative stress. One way to do this is through establishing a direct connection to the earth. This practice is known as "grounding" or "earthing." The idea behind this practice is that direct contact with Earth's surface allows you to absorb negative electrons from the earth, which can help reduce inflammation and neuter the free radicals that cause oxidative stress in the body.

Indeed, Earth's surface maintains a slight negative charge. To explain this phenomenon, I begin in the high reaches of our atmosphere.

The ionosphere is a layer of Earth's upper atmosphere, roughly between 80 km to 1,000 km (50 to 600 miles) above Earth, which is ionized by solar radiation. High-energy photons from the sun knock electrons off nitrogen and oxygen atoms at those altitudes, creating a layer of free electrons and positive ions. In addition to solar radiation, cosmic rays (high-energy particles from space) also contribute to ionizing the atmospheric gasses, leading to the formation of more charged particles.

While both positive ions and free electrons are created, the overall structure of the ionosphere tends to be net positive. In psychology, positivity is associated with lightness and negativity with heaviness. In physics, it's quite the opposite. The ionosphere is positive because electrons, which are much lighter, move freely, sometimes being lost to space or diffusing to lower altitudes while the weightier positive ions remain.

Additionally, lightning and precipitation help transfer negative charge to Earth's surface. During a thunderstorm, for example, a large amount of negative charge is carried from the clouds to the ground through lightning bolts. This is a continual process occurring all over Earth and contributing to the negative charge of Earth's surface.

Parenthetically, lightning also fixes nitrogen in the soil, where it is eventually used by plants to produce amino acids.

Earth and its atmosphere are part of a global electrical circuit. The ionosphere, with its positive charge, acts almost like a capacitor plate, while Earth's surface, with its negative charge, acts as the other plate. The atmosphere is the insulator between them. Currents flow in this circuit driven by atmospheric processes like thunderstorms and weather systems.

In the ionosphere, free electrons recombine with positive ions over time, but the continual input of energy from the sun keeps ionizing the gasses. At night, when the part of the ionosphere in shadow experiences less solar radiation, recombination reduces the ionization levels. However, even at night, cosmic rays and other sources of energy ensure that the ionosphere remains ionized, albeit at lower levels than during the day.

Both the ionosphere's positive charge and Earth's negative charge are part of a dynamic system, influenced by daily solar cycles, seasonal changes, and varying weather patterns. This system ensures that, on average, Earth maintains its slightly negative charge and the ionosphere maintains its positive charge.

Earth's surface, particularly soil and water bodies, is conductive. This conductivity allows for the free movement of charges and the maintenance of Earth's negative charge. When you "ground" or "earth" yourself by walking barefoot, for example, you are connecting to this negatively charged surface.

The theory is that through this direct contact, our bodies absorb negative ions. These negative ions are believed to neutralize free radicals, which are positively charged and can cause oxidative stress in the body.

Free radicals, as discussed in the chapter "Eating Stressed Plants," are derived from normal metabolic processes in the human body. Factories sometimes produce defective products. Our mitochondria, our energy factories, produce free radicals during the process of making ATP. Free radicals are also generated in response to external agents such as exposure to X-rays, ozone, cigarette smoking, air pollutants, and industrial chemicals. In some cases, free radicals can be useful but too many of them spell trouble.

The yang of free radicals is *yinned* by antioxidants, molecules that donate an electron to a rampaging free radical and neutralize it.

Absorbing negative ions through grounding is theorized to mimic the effect of antioxidants. The negative ion stabilizes the free radical through pairing its electron with the free radical's uncommitted electron. Yes, even free radicals, given the right conditions, will settle down and get married.

While the study samples have been small, research is supporting the health-conferring impacts of grounding. In a paper published in the *Journal of Inflammation Research*, scientists found that grounding normalized cortisol profiles, improved sleep, reduced stress levels, and lowered inflammation.[11]

The easiest way to "ground" is to simply smooch the ground with your bare feet. Just take a walk on grass, sand, or soil.

There are various other grounding systems that are available that enable contact with Earth while sleeping or sitting at a computer. These are rudimentary conductive systems in the form of sheets, mats, wrist or ankle bands, and adhesive patches that can be used inside the home or office. These applications are connected to Earth via a cord inserted into a grounded wall outlet or attached to a grounding rod placed in the soil outside. There is also footwear made by Vivobarefoot that contains a conductive rubber sole, allowing for ion absorption while still offering protection for the foot.

Even if the antioxidant benefits of grounding may be minimal, there's every reason to bury your bare feet in the warm sand or walk on the dewy grass. This simple practice is a method to rediscover the earth.

We often equate the earth with the planet that we live on. And we use the term interchangeably with culture. *The earth* has often come to mean the people on it. We surf Google "Earth" as a means to discover the targets of our wanderlust.

But humans so easily confuse the map with the territory. The earth is, of course, the soil.

We pave it over. And then bind the biomechanics of our feet in plastic and leather only to explore a digital landscape. It's no wonder we forget the true nature of the earth.

On a flat road, you might walk at a 3 miles per hour clip. But the sand slows you down and reminds you that you cannot separate the behavior and function of your own organism from the behavior and function of your environment. You are an organment, an environism.

Touching the raw earth is a reconnection with that which has sustained you. You feel into nature and its rhythm of life. It's a reminder that every molecule of your being came from the earth and someday to the earth it will return. You are part of something bigger than yourself. You are a link in the spontaneously emerging wondrous mystery of life.

THE BODY IN BALANCE

Excitatory & Inhibitory Neurotransmitters

Immersing yourself in nature often elicits a sensation of peace and tranquility. You're apt to daydream. Your thoughts may bob like Ping-Pong balls lightly atop the pond of consciousness. This feeling is sharp contrast to a mind that is racing to make connections between disparate concepts and ideas. These experiences of consciousness are chemically underwritten by molecules called neurotransmitters.

Neurotransmitters are chemical messengers released by neurons in the brain and nervous system to transmit signals between nerve cells or from neurons to muscles or glands. These marvelous little couriers are the embodiment of the ebb and flow of life. Just as waves crest and fall in the ocean, our neurotransmitters rise and recede, creating a multitude of patterns that give rise to our thoughts, feelings, and sensations.

They play a critical role in the function of the brain and the rest of the nervous system and are involved in a wide range of physiological and psychological processes, including mood, motivation, learning, memory, and movement.

There are many different types of neurotransmitters, including serotonin, dopamine, norepinephrine, acetylcholine, and gamma aminobutyric acid (GABA). Each type of neurotransmitter has a unique chemical structure and function and interacts with different receptors on the surface of target cells in order to produce specific effects.

Neurotransmitters can be broadly classified as either excitatory or inhibitory based on the effects they have on the neurons that receive them.

Excitatory neurotransmitters, such as glutamate, acetylcholine, and norepinephrine, increase the likelihood that a neuron will fire an action potential—that is, they make the neuron more likely to send a signal to other neurons. This can lead to increased activity and stimulation in the brain and nervous system.

Inhibitory neurotransmitters, such as GABA and serotonin, have the opposite effect. They decrease the likelihood that a neuron will fire an action potential, making it less likely to send a signal. This can lead to a decrease in activity and a calming effect in the brain and nervous system.

Both excitatory and inhibitory neurotransmitters are important for proper brain function and maintaining a balance between the two is critical for normal brain activity. An imbalance in the levels of these neurotransmitters has been linked to various neurological and psychiatric disorders, such as anxiety, depression, and epilepsy.

Glutamate & GABA

The two most prominent neurotransmitters in the brain are in a neural tug-of-war, or preferably, a tug of peace. One sounds like your partner's butt muscles and the other is evocative of a legendary Swedish rock band. They are the yang and yin of the brain.

Glutamate is an excitatory neurotransmitter that is involved in a wide range of processes, including learning and memory. It is often associated with activity and stimulation.

GABA, on the other hand, is an inhibitory neurotransmitter that helps to regulate brain activity by reducing neuronal excitability. It is often associated with relaxation and calmness and is thought to play a role in the regulation of anxiety and stress.

The equilibrium between neural excitation and inhibition is essential to healthy cognitive function and behavior. A brain dominated by glutamate would only be capable of exciting itself in repeated bursts of activity. Excessive amounts of glutamate can lead to overexcitation of neurons, a condition known as excitotoxicity. This overexcitation can damage or kill neurons and has been implicated in a number of neurological disorders, including epilepsy, a neurological disorder characterized by recurrent seizures.

Seizures are essentially periods of excessive and abnormal neuronal activity in the brain. In people with epilepsy, the balance between excitatory (e.g., glutamate) and inhibitory (e.g., GABA) neurotransmission is disrupted, leading to excessive neuronal activity.

Conversely, a brain dictated by GABA would be capable of only quiet whispers of activity, with little of the necessary synchronization for meaningful communication between brain areas.

Benzodiazepines are a widely used pharmaceutical that targets GABA. "Benzos," such as Valium and Xanax, are a type of tranquilizer. They were also coined "mother's little helper" by Keith Richards of The Rolling Stones. Benzos are often prescribed to help with anxiety, sleep problems, seizures, and alcohol withdrawal. These drugs work by increasing the effects of GABA in the brain.

Again, GABA is an inhibitory neurotransmitter, which means it reduces neuronal excitability and calms down brain activity. By enhancing the effects of GABA, benzodiazepines can help reduce feelings of anxiety, induce sleep, relax muscles, and prevent seizures.

Despite their effectiveness, benzodiazepines have serious downsides. They can lead to physical dependence and withdrawal symptoms if used for long periods. They can also cause drowsiness, confusion, dizziness, and impaired memory, especially at higher doses. Long-term use has been associated with an increased risk of dementia.

Healthy brain activity thrives in the middle area between these two extremes, where a balance between excitation and inhibition generates complex patterns of activity.

E/I Balance

Healthy flexible behavior and cognition depends on ebbs and flows of brain activity. Thus, the ratio between excitation and inhibition, also known as E/I balance, is a critical metric for assessing brain fitness.

Schizophrenia, for example, is concomitant with a low E/I ratio caused by feeble glutamate receptors. Autism, conversely, is associated with a high E/I ratio caused by weak GABA receptors. Even greater excesses of excitation or inhibition may result in epileptic seizures or brain coma. In fact, individuals with autism are far more likely to have epilepsy than the average person, suggesting that both autism and epilepsy are rooted in a high E/I ratio.

Neurotransmitters and the Autonomic Nervous System

There is a direct interrelationship between environmental stimuli, emotional response, neurotransmitters, and physiology.

For example, perceived threat will activate the fight-or-flight response via the amygdala and HPA axis. This sympathetic response will activate the production of epinephrine and norepinephrine which will raise heart and respiratory rate, dilate pupils, and send blood to the extremities. Norepinephrine plays a general role in deactivating the prefrontal cortex, the region of the brain implicated in executive functions, such as planning, decision-making, working memory, personality expression, moderating social behavior, and controlling certain aspects of speech and language.

Conversely, meditation, relaxing music, or certain types of breathwork can activate the parasympathetic system. This "rest and digest" state is associated with the neurotransmitter serotonin. The prefrontal cortex (PFC), the locus of reason, has a significant number of serotonin receptors and is one of the primary areas of the brain affected by serotonin. In the brain, serotonin receptors are densely located in several areas, including the cerebral cortex (which includes the PFC), the hippocampus (a key center for memory) and various other regions of the brain involved in mood regulation and cognitive function.

Both the sympathetic and parasympathetic systems have utility. Humans are justifiably willing to sacrifice a bit of upper-level reasoning when being chased by a rhino. And, of course, we need the parasympathetic system for good digestion, sleep, and immunity.

Modern culture, however, is contributing to neurotransmitter imbalances. Twenty-four-hour news and sensationalist social media preys upon our negativity biases, making us feel as if we're always under threat. From a neurotransmitter perspective, this leads to too much excitation and not enough inhibition. Once again, too much yang at the expense of yin.

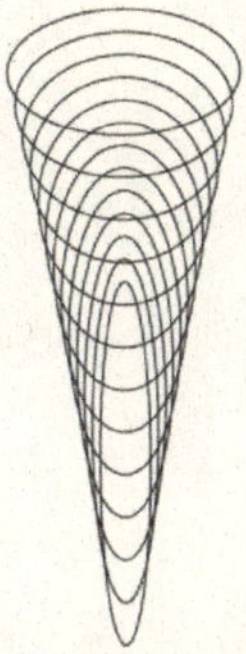

excitatory neurotransmitters are those that stimulate the brain and promote the creation of new memories, increase cognition and alertness, promote feelings of wellness, and give you energy.

GLUTAMATE: This is the most common excitatory neurotransmitter in the central nervous system. It is essential for creating memories, learning, and overall brain function.

EPINEPHRINE (ADRENALINE): This neurotransmitter affects your heart rate, muscle strength, blood pressure, and sugar metabolism, stimulating the fight-or-flight response.

NOREPINEPHRINE (NORADRENALINE): Plays a role in vigilance, attention, and mood regulation, and also stimulates the fight-or-flight response.

inhibitory neurotransmitters are those that calm the brain and help create balance by decreasing neuronal activity.

GAMMA-AMINOBUTYRIC ACID (GABA): This is the brain's main inhibitory neurotransmitter, which helps to counterbalance the excitatory (stimulating) neurotransmitters.

SEROTONIN: This neurotransmitter helps regulate mood, appetite, and sleep. While serotonin can act as both an inhibitory and excitatory neurotransmitter, it is generally considered inhibitory.

GLYCINE: An inhibitory neurotransmitter in the central nervous system, particularly in the spinal cord.

ADENOSINE: Can act as an inhibitory neurotransmitter and is involved in sleep and suppressing arousal.

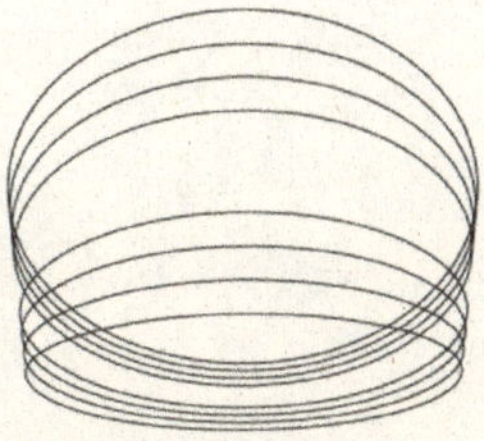

double agents

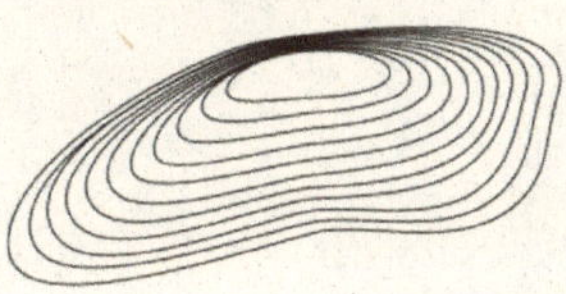

DOPAMINE: While dopamine can be both excitatory and inhibitory, its excitatory aspects help regulate movement, learning, attention, and reward-seeking behavior.

ACETYLCHOLINE: Important for muscle stimulation, memory formation, and learning. It can be both excitatory and inhibitory.

CHAPTER 20

A DAY IN THE LIFE OF GOOD STRESS

Planning is bringing the future into the present so that you can do something about it now.

— Alan Lakein

Now that we have poked and prodded at all the different protocols of Good Stress, I will provide a template for integrating them into your life. At the risk of redundancy, let me once again counsel you to ease into the practices. You want to find the edge of discomfort, not its abyss. For if the dose is too extreme, you'll never stick with it.

Here is an outline of a typical "stressful" day in my life. This schedule demonstrates how various Good Stress protocols can stack across a day. To be clear, I don't always perfectly adhere to this schedule.

Life happens. Maybe you're traveling. Maybe you're a shift worker. Maybe your regular work schedule doesn't remotely allow for this layout. Maybe it changes a bit depending on time of year. Maybe you go through a life change that derails you for an extended period. That's fine. The protocols are waiting for you to return. There's no need to be neurotic about it. In fact, orthorexia—an obsession with being healthy—is its own type of pathology. Consider this a general game plan with flexible margins.

6:00 A.M. Wake up. Drink room-temperature water. You can add some lemon if you like.

6:30 A.M. Get outside for 20 minutes. Or sit near your SAD lamp and get blue light. Combine this activity with your meditation or breathwork practice.

7:00 A.M. Have a coffee or tea. Don't add milk or sugar.

7:30 A.M. Get hot in a sauna or under a sauna blanket for 20 minutes.

8:00 A.M. Get cold in a plunge or shower for three minutes.

8:30 A.M. Go to work if you must.

11:00 A.M. "Break" fast with fiber, healthy fat, and protein.

11:30 A.M. Take a short walk—barefoot if you can.

12:00 P.M. Take five minutes to call someone you love.

2:00 P.M. Take a break and get outside without your phone. Slow down and notice things.

5:00 P.M. Move your body—preferably in nature. Mix aerobic exercise, resistance training, and flexibility work.

6:00 P.M. Make dinner with plenty of protein and vegetables, and eat it with someone if you can.

7:00 P.M. Take your last bite of food and take a short walk or do 20 push-ups.

7:15 P.M. Kick back. Read or watch a movie with your blue blockers while on the floor stretching and squatting.

9:00 P.M. Shut off all electronics. Make your bedroom cool and dark. Use only amber light. Read a book. Count your blessings. Journal your gratitudes.

9:30 P.M. Engage in some simple parasympathetic breathwork.

10:00 P.M. Nighty-night.

It's not all that stressful. It's *good* stressful.

We so often associate health with downward spirals. After four weeks of Good Stress, you will begin experiencing an upward spiral. The momentum builds atop itself. There may be no greater experience in life than witnessing your own transformation. It's completely within your grasp through doing hard things.

CONCLUSION

Living & Dying with Ease

We were all dead once. Was it so bad?

— Alan Watts

In the preceding chapters, I have made a strong case for Good Stress. Living a little more like Ffej helps the body-mind accomplish what it was designed to do: find balance.

Adopting these protocols helped me balance my blood sugar, balance my gut, balance my hormones, balance my emotional state, and even balance my social life.

But, in conclusion, I present the annoying sort of question my daughter might ask: Why?

Why is fostering balance so important? What kind of life do we really seek? What begets *true* comfort and ease?

We know bona fide comfort and ease when we taste it. It's not in the flavorless ethylene-gassed tomato from Stop & Shop. Real ease tastes like the sweet Cherokee purple tomato that bursts in your mouth—the one you grew, with a degree of inconvenience, in your own garden bed from a seedling.

Upon rigorous and honest examination, we don't want the Netflix in a pleather armchair, 72-degrees-with-a-pint-of-mint-chip-ice-cream type of comfort, even if that's occasionally delightful. Rather, we seek a life of passionate serenity. Indeed, those words at first blush seem mutually exclusive, yet we intuitively know how their marriage complement each other.

We glimpse this state of vibrant tranquility when we are deeply immersed in creative expression or collective enterprise. This feeling is often characterized by the loss of our sense of linear time, as when we're writing, playing music or sport, or deep in conversation. We move with perfect awareness of our bodies in space. We feel a sense of connection to something greater than ourselves. We have no fear. We're dancing as if we had no audience. We know without knowing. Life feels easy. We are in a flow state, our nervous system in perfect, if temporary, balance—the place on the teeter-totter when no one's feet are touching the ground.

Let me take you back to the future, to my dream in the cabin that I shared in the early pages of this tome. The year is 2088. Schuyler and I hike up to our mountain abode at 118 years old, celebrating a century together. We cook a sumptuous meal, cuddle by the fire, and equanimously float out of time, space, location, and form. We have led a life fully lived—inevitably crowded with obstacles and full of loss but without physical decrepitude, cognitive decay, and, ultimately, without the fear of death.

This is the life—and the end—we all yearn for. This is the real "ease" we seek. And while it's paradoxical that bouts of acute stress yield this ease, it's true. There are transformational health benefits to doing hard things.

The Good Stress protocols in this book, if adopted, will enhance your physical and psychological healthspan—your ability to *live* with ease. But what about death? How do we *die* with ease?

We live at a strange point along the march of evolution. By some fortuitous combination of atoms in our brains, *Homo sapiens* became conscious.

We enjoy the delight of lounging languorously sipping Sancerre with old friends. We are mesmerized by the sun dipping into a scarlet horizon. We can acknowledge our own growth—spiritual and physical—and also revel in the development of our progeny as they become our equals. We can package our thoughts and emotions in words and images such that individual perception can become collective. It's one thing to *be* happy. It's quite another thing to *know* that you are happy or sad. There is a feeling, if somewhat ineffable, of what it is like to be you. This sensation is often referred to as qualia. This phenomenon is the sunny side of consciousness.

But like a mountain, consciousness also has a shady side. We all live under the pall of knowing that everyone we love and cherish, including ourselves, is bound to die. This awareness of our own mortality elicits paroxysms of anxiety. For most of us, our inevitable demise is the ultimate and ever-present "bad" stress. And our mortality awareness has bred a hostile relationship with nature.

As a result of wrestling with our transience, we humans have spent millennia killing every creature bigger than us. Rewind 2 million years and the world was teeming with fantastic, albeit threatening beasts. Giant wombats and seven-foot flightless birds prowled Australia while rhinoceri and cave hyenas roamed Eurasia. North America boasted dire wolves and giant sloths. South America enjoyed 4,500-pound bears. Across all continents were massive, long-nosed creatures that included the notorious woolly mammoths and mastodons. Today, the remaining great beasts of Earth are largely relegated to zoos and game parks where they pose no threat. Most species of megafauna are extinct and humans are primarily to blame.

Once humans had done away with predatory macro-organisms, we turned our attention to the micro. Ever since Pasteur established germ theory in 1861, we've spent inordinate effort killing everything *smaller* than us. We can certainly celebrate the significant triumphs of antibiotics and vaccinology: 300 million people died in the 20th century from smallpox alone, and the disease killed 3 in every 10 people it infected before a vaccine was developed.[1] But, of course, as we're apt to do, humans have gone too far. Through the overapplication of antibiotics, herbicides, and pesticides, we have decimated the bacteria both in our guts and in our soil, and, in so doing, we have profoundly undermined human, plant, and planetary health.

Indeed, we mistakenly see nature as something separate from ourselves, something to be tamed and conquered. Our antagonism toward the natural world will eventually lead to our own undoing for humans co-evolved with plants, oceans, forests, animals, and prokaryotic life. We rely on each other. When a species has no predators, visible or invisible, it only has itself to fight. And, in this respect, we appear to be doing a fine job.

Our fear of death has also led to the creation of colossal myths that promise everlasting life . . . if. We are promised a rather dreary perpetuity of sitting in cold ethereal pews, chanting ecclesiastical nursery rhymes, provided that we follow the edicts and decrees of an invisible, yet oddly bearded, patriarch. This old bogey who sits in a celestial panopticon with a moral abacus monitoring our transgressions will purportedly be the arbiter of our eternal fate.

Our fear of death too often eclipses our evolutionary advantages. We are apt to abandon our neo-mammalian prefrontal cortex and turn to blind faith—belief in the absence of evidence—as a means of managing the anxiety of mortality.

Of course, our attempts to defy death pre-date the promises of dusty old Abrahamic scrolls. The Egyptians began mummifying their dead in 2600 B.C.E. The deceased were given a properly furnished tomb with all the accouterments needed for life in the afterworld.[2]

Modernity offers a different form of mummification. As a means for preserving our cadavers from decomposition, the modern West opts, unsurprisingly, for chemicals. We embalm Gramma by injecting her with formaldehyde. Further, we are the only species that hoards our dead because we think maybe, just maybe, we can cheat the mortality game.

Sometime in the 1700s, when death ceased to be the province of a man in a robe and a merlin's cap, it shifted to another man, this time in a crisp white coat. Humanity shifted its faith from the mystical to the medical, hoping the doctors would ensure everlasting life with pills and potions. Alas, the physicians only succeeded at prolonging the inevitable. Medicine provided the possibility, if chimeric, that everlasting life was in our own hands.

Walt Disney was said to be cryogenically frozen such that he could be revived when technology unlocked immortality. It turns out that this myth of "Disney on ice" was apocryphal, but it inspired scores to contemplate lives that have no end. Now, Jeff Bezos, among other fleece-vested bro-scientists, is chasing immortality, also known as escape velocity—where our organs regenerate faster than we age.

Longevity science is all the rage, bursting with esoterica from rapamycin to NAD drips, from ozone therapy to hyperbaric chambers. I'm into it . . . to a point. I wear an Oura ring, an Apple watch, and a continuous glucose monitor on my triceps. Michelle, my friendly neighborhood phlebotomist, visits every six months and draws what seems to be too much blood and, a mere three days later, 46 biomarkers appear on my phone.

But I have to ask myself: *If I were amortal and the only way I could die would be via a horrendous accident, would I ever leave my house? Would the fear of losing it all be too great?*

Of course, we all want long, healthy lives but isn't it the shadow of inevitable death itself that makes living so precious?

Yes, I want to die "young at an old age." I honestly subscribe to my mawkish dream from the early pages of this book. But part of living with ease is also dying with it. The Buddhist practice of maranasati and Stoicism's memento mori are contemplations of one's own death. Through sitting in one's transience, one may develop greater gratitude for the miracle of the next breath. Indeed, surrendering to our own mortality is perhaps the most difficult Good Stress protocol.

An essential part of this quest is reframing our relationship with nature.

Sure, our sensory instruments—our tools of conscious attention—are co-terminous with death: The irreversible cessation of circulatory, respiratory, and brain function. But what we are really is an extraordinary assembly of 7 octillion atoms—mostly oxygen, hydrogen, carbon, nitrogen, calcium, and phosphorus. All these atoms that make up the vibratory dance of life on Earth are traceable to supernovas that existed some 8 billion years ago. Under unfathomable pressure and temperatures, heavy elements were forged in the crucibles of these stars from lighter ones. Eventually, these high-mass stars became unstable and exploded, vomiting their enriched guts across the universe. These scattered elements became part of gas clouds that condensed and collapsed to form new solar systems. One of the far-flung rocks in this cosmic exercise was Earth and it contained all the elements needed for life.

Over an incomprehensible period of time, nature assembled these atoms to create leopards and woodpeckers and you and me. Some of the very same atoms that make up your physical organism also made up the Buddha, Lao Tzu, Mother Teresa, and Martin Luther King.

In fact, with each breath we take, we share an atom of oxygen with every human who has ever been born on planet Earth.

When we understand ourselves as delegated agents of this massive experiment of construction and destruction, when we feel the wonder and awe of it, it's easier to let go of the petty anxieties that we stack like masons building a brick house. A life of ease includes freedom from the anxiety of mortality. In fact, freedom from the fear of death may be the primary target of an examined life.

We spend an enormous amount of time in our brief lives extracting the bounty of nature. In death, the only polite thing to do is to flow back into it, to donate our nitrogen and carbon and hydrogen back to the soil.

A common Alan Watts refrain was, "Like the apple tree apples, the universe peoples."[3] Each one of us grows out of the world like a wave from an ocean. The great sea *waves*, expressing itself through crests of water that swell out of it, only to briefly wave at the world and then subside back into the depths. Indeed, we are each but waves in a cosmic ocean, nature's delegated adaptability, here to briefly wave at the world.

Like the ocean experiences itself as a wave, the universe experiences itself as you, here and now. Information—genetics, epigenetics, accrued experience, and knowledge—becomes briefly animated in a form you call yourself. When we cease to be animated, we once again become subsumed by the great ocean of life. Nature then selects for the best of us and reanimates another form. We come. We go.

As woo-woo as it may sound, the entirety of the universe is in us. As Watts proffered, "Your real self is the universe as centered on your organism."[4] So, on a clear night, when you go outside and behold the vast Milky Way, you can know that you are that stardust. And, in that way, you never die.

The plight of humanity is mirrored in the heavens. Like a star burns and extinguishes, so too does the life of man. The question then is: In your brief illumination, how brightly will you shine?

With a little *Good Stress*, you will light up the sky.

RESOURCES

Online Courses

Commune (onecommune.com) has the most extensive library of integrative medicine courses as well as yoga, meditation, and personal development content. Commune contributors include Dr. Mark Hyman, Dr. Sara Gottfried, Dr. Zach Bush, Dr. Gabor Maté, Dr. Casey Means, Dr. David Perlmutter, Deepak Chopra, Marianne Williamson, Alan Watts, Ram Dass, and many others.

Book Recommendations

Taoism: *Tao Te Ching* (Stephen Mitchell Translation)
Buddhism: *The Way of Zen* by Alan Watts
Physics & Spirituality: *The Tao of Physics* by Fritjof Capra
Social Science: *Sapiens & Homo Deus* by Yuval Harari
Consciousness: *Waking Up* by Sam Harris
Longevity: *Young Forever* by Dr. Mark Hyman, *Outlive* by Dr. Peter Attia
Food as Medicine: *Eat to Beat Disease* by Dr. William Li
Metabolism: *Good Energy* by Dr. Casey Means & Calley Means, *Why We Get Sick* by Dr. Ben Bikman
Epigenetics: *Younger You* by Dr. Kara Fitzgerald, *The Biology of Belief* by Dr. Bruce Lipton
Hormones: *Women, Food & Hormones* by Dr. Sara Gottfried, *Dopamine Nation* by Dr. Anna Lembke
Microbiome: *Fiber-Fueled* by Dr. Will Bulsiewicz
Brain Health: *Brain Maker* by Dr. David Perlmutter, *The End of Alzheimer's* by Dr. Dale Bredesen
Autoimmunity: *The Wahl's Protocol* by Dr. Terry Wahls, *The Autoimmunity Cure* by Dr. Sara Gottfried
Fasting: *Fast Like a Girl* by Dr. Mindy Pelz, *Fast This Way* by Dave Asprey

Ketogenic Diet: *Ketotarianism* by Dr. Will Cole
Trauma: *The Myth of Normal* by Gabor Maté, *The Body Keeps the Score* by Bessel van der Kolk
Addiction: *Recovery* by Russell Brand, *In the Realm of Hungry Ghosts* by Gabor Maté
Mental Health: *Brain Energy* by Dr. Chris Palmer
Natural Science: *The Overstory* by Richard Powers
Climate Change: *Regeneration and Drawdown* by Paul Hawken

Podcasts

The *Commune Podcast* with . . . me
The *Huberman Lab* podcast with Dr. Andrew Huberman
Making Sense with Sam Harris
The Doctor's Farmacy with Dr. Mark Hyman
Rich Roll Podcast with Rich Roll
Be Here Now podcast featuring Ram Dass, Alan Watts, and others

GLOSSARY

Jeff's Magical Mystical Medical Manifest

As I began to study human physiology, everywhere I looked I found the principles of Eastern philosophy: impermanence, interdependence, and the middle way. Through intellectual rigor, modern science was proving out what the Buddha intuited 2,500 years ago—before microscopes and germ theory.

This book bridges the medical and the mystical, the empirical and the ineffable, that which is known and that which is experienced.

Across my journey I learned this: If you are interested in the metaphysical, then immerse yourself in the study of the physical, for that is where the foundational intelligence of the universe is patterned. The micro points to the macro and back.

This glossary is a melange of West and East, modern and ancient. It's my magical medical mystical manifest. You can find an expanded version at jeffkrasno.com.

2-HOBA (2-hydroxybenzylamine): A naturally occurring phenolic compound found in certain plants. It is known for its potential antioxidant properties and may play a role in reducing oxidative stress, which is linked to various chronic diseases.

Actin: A protein that forms microfilaments and is essential for muscle contraction and cell movement.

Adiponectin: An adipokine produced by adipose tissue that enhances insulin sensitivity and has anti-inflammatory properties, with higher levels associated with reduced risk of metabolic diseases.

Adversity mimetics: Practices or interventions that simulate stress or challenges to stimulate beneficial adaptive responses in the body, similar to hormesis.

Aerobic respiration: A metabolic process in which cells produce energy (ATP) by breaking down glucose in the presence of oxygen. Aerobic respiration is the most efficient way for cells to generate energy, producing up to 36 molecules of ATP per molecule of glucose, along with water and carbon dioxide as by-products.

Amino acid: Amino acids, the building blocks of proteins, are organic compounds composed of an amino group, a carboxyl group, and a unique side chain that determines their properties. There are 20 standard amino acids that combine in various sequences to form proteins, which are essential for nearly all biological processes, including cell structure, function, and metabolism.

AMPK (AMP-activated protein kinase): An enzyme that acts as a cellular energy sensor, regulating energy balance within the cell. It is activated in response to low energy levels and works to restore energy balance by stimulating pathways that generate ATP (the cell's energy currency) and inhibiting processes that consume energy. AMPK plays a crucial role in metabolism, cell growth, and maintaining overall energy homeostasis.

Amygdala: A small, almond-shaped cluster of neurons located deep within the brain's temporal lobe. It is part of the limbic system and plays a crucial role in processing emotions, particularly fear and pleasure. The amygdala is also involved in memory formation, especially memories associated with emotional events.

Amyloid Plaques: Abnormal clusters of protein fragments that accumulate between neurons in the brain, primarily associated with Alzheimer's disease, disrupting cell communication and causing damage.

Anabolism: The metabolic process by which cells build larger, complex molecules from smaller, simpler ones, essential for growth, repair, and maintenance of tissues. Anabolism requires energy and is vital for processes such as muscle growth and cellular repair.

Anapanasati: Anapanasati, meaning "mindfulness of breathing," is a foundational meditation practice focusing on the breath to cultivate mindfulness and concentration.

Anatman: Anatman, or Anatta in Pali, is a core concept in Buddhist philosophy meaning "non-self" or "no-soul." It refers to the belief that there is no permanent, unchanging self or essence in beings. Instead, the self is seen as a collection of constantly changing physical and mental components (skandhas), emphasizing impermanence and the absence of a fixed identity.

Antibodies: Specialized proteins produced by the immune system in response to the presence of foreign substances, such as bacteria, viruses, and toxins. They bind specifically to these invaders, marking them for destruction or neutralization by other immune cells. Antibodies play a crucial role in defending the body against infections and are also used in medical diagnostics and treatments.

APOE4 allele: A variant of the APOE (apolipoprotein E) gene, which is associated with an increased risk of developing Alzheimer's disease and cardiovascular diseases.

Apolipoprotein B (ApoB): A primary protein component of lipoproteins, involved in cholesterol transport and metabolism, and serves as a key marker for assessing cardiovascular disease risk.

Apoptosis: A programmed cell death mechanism essential for maintaining cellular homeostasis and normal development, allowing for the elimination of damaged or unwanted cells without causing inflammation.

Archaea: A domain of single-celled microorganisms that are similar to bacteria but have distinct genetic and biochemical characteristics. They thrive in extreme environments such as hot springs, salt lakes, and deep-sea vents, as well as more common environments like soil and the human gut. Archaea play a key role in various ecological processes, including the carbon and nitrogen cycles.

Autoimmune diseases: Autoimmune diseases occur when the immune system mistakenly attacks the body's own cells and tissues, thinking they are foreign invaders. This can lead to inflammation and damage in various parts of the body. Common autoimmune diseases include rheumatoid arthritis, lupus, multiple sclerosis, and type 1 diabetes.

Autonomic nervous system: Regulates involuntary physiological functions, divided into sympathetic and parasympathetic systems.

Bacteroidetes: A phylum of bacteria that are predominant in the human gut microbiome. They play a crucial role in breaking down complex carbohydrates and producing short-chain fatty acids, which are beneficial for gut health. A healthy balance of Bacteroidetes is essential for proper digestion, immune function, and maintaining a healthy weight.

Bio-individualities: Refers to the concept that each person has unique nutritional, genetic, and lifestyle needs based on their individual biology and environment, and that factors such as metabolism, genetic predispositions, and personal health history influence how people respond to diets, exercise, and health interventions.

Brain-derived neurotrophic factor (BDNF): A protein that supports the survival and growth of neurons, playing a crucial role in learning, memory, and brain plasticity. Dysregulation of BDNF is associated with various neurological disorders.

BRCA1 (breast cancer 1) gene: A gene that produces a protein responsible for repairing damaged DNA, playing a crucial role in maintaining genomic stability. Mutations in the BRCA1 gene can significantly increase the risk of developing breast, ovarian, and other cancers because they impair the cell's ability to repair DNA, leading to uncontrolled cell growth.

Catabolism: The metabolic process through which complex molecules are broken down into simpler ones, releasing energy stored in the chemical bonds. This process provides energy for cellular functions and generates building blocks for anabolic processes.

Cerebral cortex: The outer layer of the brain, responsible for higher brain functions, including perception, cognition, reasoning, and voluntary motor control. The cerebral cortex plays a crucial role in complex behaviors and is essential for integrating information from various sources to produce responses.

Chromosomes: Thread-like structures composed of DNA and proteins found in the nucleus of most living cells. They carry genetic information in the form of genes and are responsible for the inheritance of traits from one generation to the next.

***Clostridium difficile*:** A type of bacteria that can cause severe diarrhea and inflammation of the colon, known as colitis. It often occurs after the use of antibiotics, which disrupt the normal gut microbiota and allow C. difficile to proliferate. Infection can lead to symptoms such as abdominal pain, fever, and dehydration and can be life-threatening if not treated properly.

Coincidentia oppositorum: A Latin term meaning the "coincidence of opposites," referring to the concept that contradictory or opposing elements can coexist and be reconciled within a higher unity or truth. This idea is prominent in philosophy and theology and is often associated with the works of philosopher Nicholas of Cusa and other mystical traditions.

Continuous partial attention: A state of divided attention where a person constantly monitors multiple information sources, often facilitated by technology.

Contractile proteins: Proteins involved in muscle contraction and movement. The primary contractile proteins are actin and myosin, which interact to generate the force needed for muscle fibers to contract. These proteins are essential not only in skeletal muscle function but also in the movement of cells and the maintenance of cellular shape.

Cortisol: A steroid hormone produced by the adrenal glands in response to stress and low blood-glucose levels. It is known as the body's primary stress hormone and plays a vital role in regulating metabolism, reducing inflammation, and assisting with memory formation.

Counterregulatory molecules: Substances, such as hormones or proteins, that act to balance or counteract the effects of other molecules within the body to maintain homeostasis. For example, in response to low blood sugar, counterregulatory hormones like glucagon and adrenaline increase blood glucose levels, opposing the action of insulin, which lowers blood sugar.

C-reactive protein (CRP):A substance produced by the liver in response to inflammation. Elevated levels of CRP in the blood are a marker of acute inflammation and can indicate conditions such as infection, autoimmune disorders, or cardiovascular disease.

Cytoplasm: The jelly-like substance within a cell, enclosed by the cell membrane, and excluding the nucleus. It contains various organelles, such as mitochondria and ribosomes, and is the site of numerous biochemical processes essential for the cell's survival and function, including protein synthesis, cell division, and metabolic reactions.

Cytosine nucleotide: A building block of DNA and RNA that consists of the nitrogenous base cytosine, a sugar molecule (deoxyribose in DNA or ribose in RNA), and a phosphate group. In DNA, cytosine pairs with guanine to form the rungs of the double helix structure. Cytosine nucleotides are essential for encoding genetic information and play a role in gene expression and regulation.

DNA (deoxyribonucleic acid): The molecule that carries genetic instructions necessary for the growth, development, and reproduction of all living organisms, composed of nucleotides arranged in a double helix structure.

Dysbiosis: An imbalance in the microbial communities within the body, particularly in the gut. This disruption can lead to an overgrowth of harmful bacteria and a reduction in beneficial microbes, affecting digestion, immune function, and overall health. Dysbiosis has been linked to conditions such as irritable bowel syndrome (IBS), inflammatory bowel disease (IBD), and metabolic disorders.

Ectopic fat: Fat that is stored in abnormal locations within the body, such as in organs like the liver, heart, muscles, and pancreas. Unlike subcutaneous fat, ectopic fat can interfere with organ function and is linked to conditions like insulin resistance, type 2 diabetes, and cardiovascular disease.

Endocrine disruptor: A chemical substance that can interfere with the endocrine (hormonal) system, affecting the body's development, reproduction, neurological function, and immune response. Common sources include pesticides, plastics, and personal care products.

Endocrine response: The physiological reactions initiated by hormones released into the bloodstream by endocrine glands in response to internal or external stimuli, regulating various bodily functions such as metabolism and stress responses.

Endothelium: A thin layer of cells lining blood vessels, playing a crucial role in vascular health.

Endotoxemia: Endotoxemia is a condition characterized by the presence of endotoxins in the bloodstream, which can trigger an inflammatory response and lead to symptoms such as fever and septic shock.

Endotoxins: Toxic components found in the outer membrane of certain bacteria. They are released when the bacteria die and disintegrate, triggering strong immune responses in the host.

Enzymes: Biological catalysts that speed up chemical reactions in the body without being consumed in the process. They play essential roles in various biochemical processes, including digestion, metabolism, and DNA replication. Each enzyme is specific to a particular reaction or type of reaction, allowing the body to efficiently regulate and perform complex biochemical functions.

Epigenetics: The study of changes in gene expression that do not involve alterations to the underlying DNA sequence. These changes can be influenced by environmental factors, such as diet, stress, and toxins, and can affect how genes are turned on or off.

Epigenome: The complete set of epigenetic modifications on the genetic material of a cell, influencing gene expression without altering the underlying DNA sequence.

Epithelial wall: The layer of epithelial cells that line organs and structures within the body, such as the gut, lungs, and blood vessels. It acts as a protective barrier, regulates the absorption of nutrients and water, and prevents the entry of harmful substances and pathogens. The integrity of the epithelial wall is essential for maintaining overall health and preventing disease.

***Escherichia coli*:** A diverse group of bacteria that normally reside in the intestines of humans and animals. While most strains are harmless and play a role in maintaining gut health, some can cause serious foodborne illness. Pathogenic strains are often transmitted through contaminated food or water.

Etiology: The study of the causes or origins of diseases and medical conditions. It involves identifying factors such as pathogens, genetics, environmental influences, and lifestyle choices that contribute to the development of a disease.

Eustress: A positive form of stress that can motivate and enhance performance or well-being. It occurs in situations perceived as challenging but manageable and beneficial, such as starting a new job, exercising, or achieving a goal. Eustress promotes personal growth and resilience, in contrast to distress, which can lead to anxiety and negative health outcomes.

Euthymia: A state of mental well-being characterized by stable mood and emotional balance, free from depressive or manic episodes.

Exposome: Refers to the totality of environmental exposures individuals experience throughout their lifetime, from conception onwards. It encompasses all external factors—such as air quality, diet, lifestyle, and social environment—as well as internal biological responses to these exposures, influencing health and disease outcomes.

Firmicutes: A phylum of bacteria commonly found in the human gut and other environments. They are involved in the fermentation of dietary fibers into short-chain fatty acids, which provide energy and support gut health. The balance of Firmicutes in the microbiome can influence metabolism, immune function, and overall health.

Fisetin: A flavonoid found in various fruits and vegetables, including strawberries, apples, and onions. It is recognized for its antioxidant properties and potential health benefits, which include anti-inflammatory effects, neuroprotective properties, and the ability to enhance cognitive function.

Free radicals: Highly reactive atoms or molecules that contain unpaired electrons, causing cellular damage and contributing to aging and diseases when produced in excess.

GABA (gamma-aminobutyric acid): The primary inhibitory neurotransmitter in the central nervous system. It reduces neuronal excitability by binding to GABA receptors, leading to the opening of ion channels and a decrease in the likelihood of neurons firing.

Ghrelin: A hormone produced primarily in the stomach that stimulates appetite and promotes food intake. It is often referred to as the "hunger hormone" because its levels increase before meals and decrease after eating. Ghrelin also plays a role in regulating energy balance, metabolism, and the release of growth hormone.

Glutamate: The most abundant excitatory neurotransmitter in the brain, playing a critical role in cognitive functions such as learning and memory. It is involved in synaptic plasticity, which is essential for neural communication and adaptation. Dysregulation of glutamate signaling is associated with various neurological and psychiatric disorders, including epilepsy, schizophrenia, and Alzheimer's disease.

Glycolysis: The metabolic pathway that converts glucose into pyruvate, producing energy in the form of ATP.

Gut epithelium cells: Specialized epithelial cells that form a barrier on the surface of the intestines. They facilitate nutrient absorption, secrete mucus to protect the gut lining, and play a crucial role in immune defense by preventing the entry of harmful substances and pathogens.

Gut flora: Gut flora, also known as gut microbiota, refers to the diverse community of microorganisms, including bacteria, viruses, fungi, and other microbes, residing in the gastrointestinal tract. These microbes play a vital role in digestion, nutrient absorption, immune function, and overall gut health.

Gut microbial phyla: The major classifications of bacteria that inhabit the human gastrointestinal tract. The most dominant phyla are Firmicutes and Bacteroidetes, which play key roles in digesting food, producing essential nutrients, and maintaining a balanced immune system. Other important phyla include Actinobacteria and Proteobacteria, each contributing to gut health and overall well-being.

HBB gene: Provides instructions for making beta-globin, a key component of hemoglobin, the protein in red blood cells that carries oxygen throughout the body.

HDL (high-density lipoprotein): Helps transport cholesterol to the liver for excretion.

***Helicobacter pylori*:** A type of bacteria that infects the stomach lining and is a common cause of peptic ulcers and chronic gastritis. It can disrupt the protective mucus layer of the stomach, leading to inflammation and damage to the stomach lining.

Hematopoietic stem cells: Multipotent stem cells found in the bone marrow that give rise to all types of blood cells, including red blood cells, white blood cells, and platelets. They play a critical role in the body's ability to replenish and maintain the blood system.

Hippocampus: A region of the brain involved in memory formation and spatial navigation.

Holotropic breathwork: A therapeutic breathing practice developed by Stanislav Grof that uses accelerated breathing patterns to induce altered states of consciousness.

Homeostasis: The process by which living organisms maintain a stable internal environment despite external changes. This balance is crucial for proper functioning and involves the regulation of factors like temperature, pH, and electrolyte levels.

Hominin: A group of species that includes modern humans (*Homo sapiens*) and our closest extinct relatives, such as *Australopithecus* and *Homo neanderthalensis*. Hominins are characterized by traits like bipedalism and larger brain sizes compared to other primates, reflecting evolutionary adaptations over millions of years.

Hormesis: A biological phenomenon where exposure to a low dose of a harmful agent or stressor stimulates beneficial adaptive responses in cells and organisms, improving health and stress resistance.

HPA axis: The HPA (hypothalamic-pituitary-adrenal) axis is a complex network of interactions among the hypothalamus, pituitary gland, and adrenal glands. It regulates the body's response to stress by controlling the release of cortisol and other hormones and plays a key role in maintaining homeostasis.

Hydroxyl radical: A highly reactive free radical formed from the combination of hydrogen and oxygen, playing a significant role in oxidative stress and cellular damage.

Hyperinsulinemia: A condition characterized by excessively high levels of insulin in the blood. It is often associated with insulin resistance and can lead to type 2 diabetes, obesity, and cardiovascular disease.

Hypermethylation: An increase in the addition of methyl groups to specific regions of DNA that can lead to the silencing of genes, including tumor suppressor genes, preventing them from carrying out their normal function. Hypermethylation is associated with various diseases, including cancer, as it can disrupt normal cellular processes and promote uncontrolled cell growth.

Hyperplasia: A physiological process characterized by an increase in the number of cells in a tissue or organ, leading to its enlargement. This process can occur in response to various stimuli, such as hormonal changes or injury, and is often a normal adaptive mechanism.

Hypocapnia: A condition characterized by abnormally low levels of carbon dioxide in the blood, often resulting from hyperventilation.

Hypoxia: A condition characterized by insufficient oxygen supply to the tissues, which can lead to symptoms such as shortness of breath and fatigue.

Indra's Net: A metaphorical concept in Mahayana Buddhism and Hinduism that illustrates the interconnectedness and interdependence of all things in the universe. It is depicted as a vast, cosmic net with a multifaceted jewel at each intersection, where each jewel reflects all the others, symbolizing how every entity is connected in an intricate, infinite web of existence.

Insulin Resistance: A condition where the body's cells do not respond effectively to insulin, leading to elevated blood sugar levels. It is often associated with obesity, type 2 diabetes, and metabolic syndrome.

Insulin-like growth factor 1 (IGF-1): A protein hormone produced in the liver that promotes cell growth and development in response to growth hormone stimulation. It plays a key role in anabolic processes and is associated with muscle growth and repair.

Interleukin-6 and TNF-alpha: Cytokines involved in inflammation and immune responses, often elevated in various diseases.

Intestinal permeability: Often gruesomely nicknamed "leaky gut," this is a condition in which the lining of the small intestine becomes damaged, allowing undigested food particles, toxins, and bacteria to pass through the intestinal wall into the bloodstream, which can trigger immune responses and inflammation.

Jiji Muge: A concept in Japanese Zen Buddhism that expresses the boundless interpenetration and interconnectedness of all phenomena. It suggests that every element of the universe is in a dynamic relationship with every other element, without any barriers or obstructions. This idea reflects the ultimate non-dual reality where all distinctions dissolve.

Kaempferol: A flavonoid found in various plants, including kale, spinach, and tea. Known for its antioxidant and anti-inflammatory properties, kaempferol is associated with several health benefits, including potential anti-cancer effects, improved cardiovascular health, and enhanced immune function.

Karuna: A Sanskrit term for "compassion," indicating empathy for the suffering of others.

Krebs cycle: A series of biochemical reactions that occur in the mitochondria, responsible for producing energy through the oxidation of acetyl-CoA.

Kula: In Sanskrit, the term *kula* refers to a community, clan, or family. In spiritual contexts, it can also refer to a group of devotees or followers of a particular spiritual path or teacher.

Lactobacillus: A genus of beneficial bacteria commonly found in the human gut, mouth, and female reproductive tract, as well as in fermented foods like yogurt and sauerkraut. Lactobacillus species are often used as probiotics to support digestive health, boost immunity, and restore balance to the gut microbiome.

LDL (low-density lipoprotein) particles: Lipoproteins that carry cholesterol through the bloodstream and are associated with an increased risk of cardiovascular diseases when elevated.

Leptin: A hormone produced by fat cells that helps regulate energy balance by inhibiting hunger. It signals the brain to reduce appetite and increase energy expenditure when fat stores are sufficient. Dysregulation of leptin signaling can lead to obesity and other metabolic disorders.

Limbic system: A complex set of structures in the brain that plays a crucial role in emotion, behavior, motivation, long-term memory, and olfaction. Key components include the hippocampus, amygdala, and hypothalamus, which work together to regulate emotional responses and help form memories.

Luteolin: A flavonoid present in many herbs, fruits, and vegetables. It is known for its antioxidant and anti-inflammatory properties, and research suggests it may have potential benefits in protecting against certain diseases, including cancer and neurodegenerative disorders.

Macrophage: A type of white blood cell that plays a crucial role in the immune system by engulfing and digesting cellular debris and pathogens, as well as regulating immune responses through cytokine production.

Metabolic Dysfunction: A condition where the body's normal metabolic processes are disrupted, leading to issues like insulin resistance, high blood sugar, abnormal cholesterol levels, and increased fat around the waist. It often contributes to diseases like type 2 diabetes, cardiovascular disease, and obesity.

Methyl Group: A chemical group consisting of one carbon atom bonded to three hydrogen atoms, represented as $-CH_3$. It is commonly found in organic molecules and plays a key role in many biochemical processes, including DNA methylation, where it is added to DNA to regulate gene expression.

Microbiota: The community of microorganisms, including bacteria, fungi, viruses, and archaea, that live in and on the human body, particularly in the gut. These microbial communities play essential roles in digestion, immune function, and overall health.

Mitobiogenesis: The process of creating new mitochondria within a cell, essential for maintaining cellular energy production and responding to increased energy demands.

Mitochondria: Organelles within cells that generate most of the cell's energy through the process of oxidative phosphorylation. Often referred to as the "powerhouses" of the cell, they also play roles in regulating cellular metabolism, signaling, and apoptosis (cell death).

mTOR (mechanistic Target of Rapamycin): A protein kinase that regulates cell growth, proliferation, metabolism, and survival. It functions as part of two complexes, mTORC1 and mTORC2, and plays a key role in responding to nutrient availability, energy status, and other cellular signals.

Mudita: A Pali term for "sympathetic joy," indicating joy in the happiness of others.

Myofilament: A filament of myofibrils, composed of proteins such as actin and myosin, that are responsible for muscle contraction.

Myokines: Cytokines or peptides produced by muscle cells that have autocrine, paracrine, or endocrine effects on various tissues.

Myosin: A motor protein that interacts with actin to cause muscle contraction.

N.E.A.T. (non-exercise activity thermogenesis): The energy expended for all activities not related to sleeping, eating, or sports.

NAD+ (nicotinamide adenine dinucleotide): A vital coenzyme found in all living cells, essential for redox reactions in metabolism and involved in DNA repair and cellular signaling.

Neurotransmitter: A chemical messenger that transmits signals across a synapse from one neuron (nerve cell) to another or to a target cell, such as a muscle or gland cell.

Neutrophils: A type of white blood cell and a key component of the innate immune system, responsible for rapidly responding to infections, particularly bacterial, by engulfing and digesting pathogens.

Nicotinamide mononucleotide (NMN): A nucleotide that serves as a precursor to NAD+, with potential health benefits and applications in aging research.

Nirvana: A central concept in Buddhism that refers to the ultimate state of liberation and freedom from suffering, desire, and the cycle of birth and rebirth (samsara).

NK Cells (Natural Killer Cells): A type of white blood cell that plays a crucial role in the immune system's defense against tumors and viral infections.

Non-redundant genes: Genes that perform unique and essential functions in an organism, with no other genes capable of compensating for their loss.

Nucleotide: A nucleotide is the basic building block of nucleic acids, such as DNA and RNA. It consists of three components: a nitrogenous base (adenine, thymine, cytosine, guanine, or uracil), a five-carbon sugar (deoxyribose in DNA or ribose in RNA), and one or more phosphate groups.

Oleuropein: A bitter phenolic compound found in olive leaves and olive oil, known for its antioxidant and anti-inflammatory properties.

Organelles: Specialized structures within a cell that perform distinct functions necessary for the cell's survival and proper functioning. Examples include the nucleus (which houses genetic material), mitochondria (responsible for energy production), and the endoplasmic reticulum (involved in protein and lipid synthesis).

Orthorexia: An eating disorder characterized by an excessive preoccupation with healthy eating and the avoidance of foods deemed unhealthy or impure. Individuals with orthorexia may become overly restrictive in their dietary choices, leading to nutritional deficiencies and social isolation.

Paleolithic genome: The genetic makeup of humans during the Paleolithic era (from about 2.5 million to 10,000 years ago), reflecting the evolutionary adaptations of early hunter-gatherers.

Parasympathetic breath: A breathing technique designed to activate the parasympathetic nervous system, promoting relaxation and reducing stress.

Peptide hormone: A type of hormone composed of amino acids arranged in a chain. These hormones, such as insulin and glucagon, regulate a variety of physiological processes including metabolism, growth, and development.

Peripheral nervous system: The part of the nervous system outside the brain and spinal cord.

Phytoncides: Antimicrobial compounds released by plants that help protect them from pathogens and insects. These substances have been shown to have beneficial effects on human health, including reducing stress, enhancing immune function, and promoting overall well-being.

Phytonutrients: Naturally occurring compounds found in plants that contribute to their color, flavor, and disease resistance. They provide health benefits to humans, including antioxidant, anti-inflammatory, and immune-boosting effects.

Piceatannol: Piceatannol is a natural polyphenolic compound structurally similar to resveratrol, found in various plants, including grapes and berries. It is known for its antioxidant properties and potential health benefits.

Pineal gland: The pineal gland is a small, pea-shaped endocrine gland located in the brain that produces and secretes the hormone melatonin, which regulates sleep-wake cycles and circadian rhythms.

Pleiotropic: Referring to a phenomenon where a single gene influences multiple traits or biological functions.

Polyphenols: Naturally occurring compounds found in plants, known for their antioxidant properties and potential health benefits, including reducing the risk of chronic diseases.

Pranayama: A practice in yoga that involves the regulation and control of the breath. It is derived from the Sanskrit words *prana* (life force or breath) and *ayama* (extension or control) and considered a key aspect of yogic discipline for physical and spiritual well-being.

Pratityasamutpāda: A fundamental Buddhist concept that explains the interconnectedness and conditionality of all phenomena. This principle is central to understanding the nature of suffering and the cycle of birth, death, and rebirth (samsara), highlighting that all experiences are interdependent and transient.

Prefrontal Cortex: The part of the frontal lobes involved in complex cognitive behavior and decision-making.

Prokaryotes: Single-celled organisms, including bacteria and archaea, that lack a membrane-bound nucleus and other organelles. Their genetic material is contained in a single, circular chromosome located in the cell cytoplasm.

Proprioception: The body's ability to sense its position, movement, and orientation in space. It involves specialized receptors in the muscles, tendons, and joints that provide feedback to the brain about the position and movement of different body parts. This sense allows for coordinated movement and balance.

Protein-coding genes: Segments of DNA that contain the instructions for synthesizing proteins. These genes are transcribed into messenger RNA (mRNA), which is then translated into a specific sequence of amino acids to form a protein.

Pyruvate: A key intermediate in several metabolic pathways. It is the end product of glycolysis, where one molecule of glucose is broken down to form two molecules of pyruvate. Pyruvate can be further metabolized to produce energy through the citric acid cycle (aerobic respiration) or converted into lactate or ethanol under anaerobic conditions.

Quercetin: A flavonoid found in many fruits, vegetables, and grains, known for its antioxidant properties.

Rasmussen's Encephalitis: A rare, chronic inflammatory brain disorder, mainly affecting children. It causes frequent seizures, one-sided body weakness (hemiparesis), cognitive decline, and speech problems.

Red blood cells: Cells in the blood that carry oxygen from the lungs to the rest of the body and return carbon dioxide to the lungs for exhalation. They contain hemoglobin, a protein that binds oxygen, and have a characteristic biconcave shape.

Resistin: An adipokine linked to insulin resistance, produced by adipose tissue, and associated with obesity and metabolic syndrome.

Resveratrol: A polyphenolic compound found in red wine, grapes, berries, and peanuts, known for its antioxidant properties.

Ribosomes: Small, complex molecular machines found within all living cells that are responsible for synthesizing proteins. They translate messenger RNA (mRNA) sequences into amino acid chains, forming proteins based on the genetic instructions provided by the cell's DNA.

Rutin: A flavonoid glycoside found in various plants, including buckwheat and citrus fruits. It is recognized for its antioxidant properties and potential benefits in strengthening blood vessels and reducing inflammation.

Salidroside: A natural phenolic compound primarily found in the herb *Rhodiola rosea*. It is known for its adaptogenic properties, which may help the body adapt to stress and improve overall resilience.

Samadhi: A state of deep meditation and spiritual absorption, representing unity with the object of meditation.

Serotonin: A neurotransmitter that plays a key role in regulating mood, emotions, sleep, and appetite. Serotonin levels can be influenced by diet, exercise, and exposure to sunlight, and imbalances in serotonin are linked to mood disorders such as depression and anxiety.

Single nucleotide polymorphisms (SNPs): Variations in a single nucleotide base in the DNA sequence among individuals. These genetic differences can occur within genes or in the non-coding regions of the genome.

Single-celled microbes: Microorganisms consisting of only one cell that perform all the necessary functions of life within that single unit. These include bacteria, archaea, protozoa, and some types of fungi and algae. Single-celled microbes play critical roles in ecosystems, such as decomposing organic material, cycling nutrients, and forming the basis of food webs.

Sirtuins: A family of proteins that function as NAD^+-dependent deacetylases, involved in regulating cellular processes such as metabolism, stress response, and aging.

Somatic nervous system: A component of the peripheral nervous system responsible for voluntary movements.

Stoneman Syndrome: A rare genetic disorder in which soft tissues progressively turn into bone, restricting movement.

Storage proteins: Proteins that serve as reserves of amino acids and other essential nutrients for later use. Examples include casein in milk, which provides amino acids to growing mammals, and gluten in wheat, which stores nutrients for seed germination.

Structural proteins: Proteins that provide support, strength, and shape to cells and tissues in the body. Examples include collagen, which provides tensile strength to skin and bones, and keratin, which is found in hair and nails.

Sulforaphane: A bioactive compound found in cruciferous vegetables, particularly in broccoli, Brussels sprouts, and kale. It is recognized for its potential antioxidant and anti-cancer properties, as it may help activate detoxification enzymes and protect against oxidative stress.

Suprachiasmatic nucleus (SCN): A small group of neurons located in the hypothalamus that serves as the primary circadian clock in the body, regulating sleep-wake cycles and various physiological processes in response to light and dark.

Sympathetic nervous system: Part of the autonomic nervous system that prepares the body for stress responses, increasing heart rate and blood flow.

Tao: A central concept in Chinese philosophy and religion, particularly in Taoism. It translates to "the Way" or "the Path" and refers to the fundamental principle that underlies and unites the universe.

Tau proteins: A family of proteins that stabilize microtubules in neuronal cells. They are crucial for maintaining neuronal structure, and their dysfunction is linked to neurodegenerative diseases, such as Alzheimer's.

Thermoneutrality: The state in which an organism maintains a stable internal body temperature without expending energy on thermoregulation. In this state, the temperature of the surrounding environment is optimal for the organism, allowing it to maintain homeostasis without the need for metabolic heat production or heat loss mechanisms.

Transport proteins: Proteins that move molecules and ions across cell membranes or throughout the body. They play a vital role in regulating the internal environment of cells and organisms by facilitating the transport of substances such as oxygen, nutrients, and waste products.

Tummo: A Tibetan Buddhist meditation practice that focuses on generating inner heat and achieving a heightened state of awareness and spiritual insight.

Ubuntu: An African philosophical concept that emphasizes the interconnectedness and shared humanity of all people. Often translated as "I am because we are," it underscores the belief that an individual's well-being and identity are deeply tied to the well-being of others and the community.

Vasoconstriction: The physiological process in which blood vessels constrict, reducing blood flow and increasing blood pressure, often in response to stress or low blood volume.

Vestibular system: A complex sensory system located in the inner ear that helps regulate balance, spatial orientation, and coordination of movement.

Visceral fat: A type of body fat stored within the abdominal cavity, surrounding vital organs such as the liver, pancreas, and intestines. High levels of visceral fat are associated with increased risk of serious health conditions, including heart disease, type 2 diabetes, and metabolic syndrome.

VO_2 max: The maximum rate of oxygen consumption measured during incremental exercise, reflecting aerobic fitness.

White blood cells (leukocytes): A vital part of the immune system, helping the body to fight infections and other diseases. They circulate in the blood and lymphatic system, identifying and neutralizing foreign invaders such as bacteria, viruses, and fungi.

Wim Hof method: A breathing and meditation technique developed by Wim Hof, combining specific breathing exercises, cold exposure, and meditation.

Xenohormetins: Compounds derived from dietary sources or environmental factors that can induce a stress response in cells, leading to protective adaptations. These substances may mimic the effects of mild stress, promoting resilience and potentially benefiting health through mechanisms similar to hormesis.

Yin-yang: A fundamental concept in Chinese philosophy and Taoism that represents the duality and interconnectedness of opposing forces in the universe.

ENDNOTES

Introduction

1. O'Hearn et al., "Trends and Disparities in Cardiometabolic Health among U.S. Adults, 1999–2018," *Journal of the American College of Cardiology* 80, no. 2 (July 2022): 138–51, https://doi.org/10.1016/j.jacc.2022.04.046.

Chapter 1

1. "About Chronic Diseases," Centers for Disease Control and Prevention, n.d., https://www.cdc.gov/chronic-disease/about/index.html.
2. "About Chronic Diseases," Centers for Disease Control and Prevention.
3. "Get the Facts on Healthy Aging," National Council on Aging, August 16, 2024, https://www.ncoa.org/article/get-the-facts-on-healthy-aging/.
4. "Chronic Disease Facts and Statistics," Centers for Disease Control and Prevention, last updated July 7, 2023, https://www.cdc.gov/chronic-disease /data-research/facts-stats/index.html; Reuters, "U.S. Healthcare Spending Rises to $4.8 Trillion in 2023, Outpacing GDP," U.S. News, June 12, 2024, https://money.usnews.com/investing/news/articles/2024-06-12/u-s -healthcare-spending-rises-to-4-8-trillion-in-2023-outpacing-gdp.
5. Steve Davis, "The $12 Trillion Question: What Will Health Spending Look like in 2040?," Deloitte United States, March 9, 2021, https://www2.deloitte. com/us/en/blog/health-care-blog/2021/the-12-trillion-dollar-question-what -will-health-spending-look-like-in-2040.html.
6. "Adult Obesity Facts," Centers for Disease Control and Prevention, last updated May 17, 2022, https://www.cdc.gov/obesity/data/adult.html; "Overweight & Obesity Statistics," National Institute of Diabetes and Digestive and Kidney Diseases, last updated August 2022, https://www .niddk.nih.gov/health-information/health-statistics/overweight-obesity.
7. "National Diabetes Statistics Report, 2020: Estimates of Diabetes and Its Burden in the United States," Centers for Disease Control and Prevention, last updated August 28, 2020, https://www.cdc.gov/diabetes/data/statistics -report/index.html.
8. "Prediabetes: Could It Be You? Infographic," Centers for Disease Control and Prevention, n.d., https://www.cdc.gov/diabetes/communication-resources /prediabetes-statistics.html.

Chapter 4

1. Robin Lovell-Badge, "Life Span of Human Cells Defined: Most Cells Are Younger Than the Individual," Times Higher Education (THE), August 12, 2005, https://www.timeshighereducation.com/news/life-span-of-human -cells-defined-most-cells-are-younger-than-the-individual/198208.article.

Chapter 5

1. Ron Sender, Shai Fuchs, and Ron Milo, "Revised Estimates for the Number of Human and Bacteria Cells in the Body," *PLOS Biology* 14, no. 8 (August 19, 2016), https://doi.org/10.1371/journal.pbio.1002533.
2. "Human Genomic Variation," National Human Genome Research Institute, https://www.genome.gov/dna-day/15-ways/human-genomic-variation.

3. Qin et al., "A Human Gut Microbial Gene Catalogue Established by Metagenomic Sequencing," *Nature* 464, no. 7285 (March 4, 2010): 59–65, https://doi.org/10.1038/nature08821.
4. "The Human Genome Project Completion: Frequently Asked Questions," National Human Genome Research Institute, https://www.genome.gov/11006943/human-genome-project-completion-frequently-asked-questions/.

Chapter 6

1. The French–Italian Public Consortium for Grapevine Genome Characterization, "The Grapevine Genome Sequence Suggests Ancestral Hexaploidization in Major Angiosperm Phyla," *Nature* 449, no. 7161 (August 26, 2007): 463–67, https://doi.org/10.1038/nature06148.
2. International Human Genome Sequencing Consortium, "Finishing the Euchromatic Sequence of the Human Genome," *Nature* 431, no. 7011 (October 21, 2004): 931–45, https://doi.org/10.1038/nature03001; "The Human Genome Project." National Human Genome Research Institute, Genome.gov, updated August 24, 2022, https://www.genome.gov/human-genome-project.
3. Corder et al., "Gene Dose of Apolipoprotein e Type 4 Allele and the Risk of Alzheimer's Disease in Late Onset Families," *Science* 261, no. 5123 (August 13, 1993): 921–23, https://doi.org/10.1126/science.8346443; Fortea et al., "APOE4 Homozygosity Represents a Distinct Genetic Form of Alzheimer's Disease," *Nature Medicine* 30, no. 5 (May 2024): 1284–91, https://doi.org/10.1038/s41591-024-02931-w.
4. Esteller et al. "Hypermethylation-Associated Inactivation of the Cellular Retinoic Acid Binding Protein 1 Gene in Human Cancer," *Oncogene* 19, no. 3 (October 15, 2002): 404–409, https://pubmed.ncbi.nlm.nih.gov/12384555; Stephen B. Baylin and Peter A. Jones, "A Decade of Exploring the Cancer Epigenome — Biological and Translational Implications," *Nature Reviews Cancer* 11, no. 10 (September 23, 2011): 726–34, https://doi.org/10.1038/nrc3130.

Chapter 7

1. "What Is a Normal Respiratory Rate?" American Thoracic Society, ATS.org, https://www.thoracic.org/patients/patient-resources/resources/adult-rr.pdf.
2. "What Your Heart Rate Is Telling You," American Heart Association, Heart.org, updated October 5, 2022, https://www.heart.org/en/healthy-living/fitness/fitness-basics/target-heart-rates.
3. Amar Singh, "The Liver and Blood Glucose Levels," Diabetes.co.uk, January 15, 2019, https://www.diabetes.co.uk/body/liver-and-blood-glucose-levels.html.
4. Sophie Cousins, "The Great Puberty Shift," *The Lancet* 404, no. 10452 (August 2024): 511–12, https://doi.org/10.1016/s0140-6736(24)01640-4; Robin McKie, "Onset of Puberty in Girls Has Fallen by Five Years since 1920," The Guardian, October 20, 2012, https://www.theguardian.com/society/2012/oct/21/puberty-adolescence-childhood-onset.
5. American Academy of Pediatrics; Committee on Adolescence; American College of Obstetricians and Gynecologists; Committee on Adolescent Health Care, "Menstruation in Girls and Adolescents: Using the Menstrual Cycle as a Vital Sign," *Pediatrics* 118, no. 5 (November 1, 2006): 2245–50, https://doi.org/10.1542/peds.2006-2481.

Chapter 8

1. "EPA Report on the Environment: Indoor Air Quality," Environmental Protection Agency, updated July 8, 2024, https://www.epa.gov/report-environment/indoor-air-quality.

Chapter 9

1. "Pranayama," Ekhart Yoga, October 5, 2023, https://www.ekhartyoga.com/resources/styles/pranayama.
2. F. Max Müller, trans., *The Upanishads, Part I* (Mineola, NY: Dover Publications, 1962).
3. "Exploring the Ancient Roots and Modern Revival of Cold Water Therapy," Tundra Tribe, n.d., https://tundratribe.com/blogs/ways-of-wellness-by-tundra-tribe/exploring-the-ancient-roots-and-modern-revival-of-cold-water-therapy.; "History of Sweating," MySauna, n.d., https://mysauna.info/en/about-sauna/history-of-sweating.
4. Ma et al., "The Development of Traditional Chinese Medicine," *Journal of Traditional Chinese Medical Sciences* 8 (November 2021), https://doi.org/10.1016/j.jtcms.2021.11.002.

Chapter 10

1. Muhammad Tufail Ansari, trans., *Sunan Ibn Majah*: *Book of Fasting* (Riyadh: Darussalam Publishers, 2007).
2. Jalal al-Din Al-Suyuti, *The Book of Fasting: Guidance on the Sunnah of the Prophet Muhammad* (Cairo: Dar al-Kutub al-Ilmiyya, 1997).
3. "Figs, Dried, Uncooked," U.S. Department of Agriculture, https://fdc.nal.usda.gov/food-details/746768/nutrients.
4. Oda et al., "Loss of Urate Oxidase Activity in Hominoids and Its Evolutionary Implications," *Molecular Biology and Evolution* 19, no. 5 (May 1, 2002): 640–53, https://doi.org/10.1093/oxfordjournals.molbev.a004123.; Johnson et al., "Hypothesis: Could Excessive Fructose Intake and Uric Acid Cause Type 2 Diabetes?," *Endocrine Reviews* 30, no. 1 (January 16, 2009): 96–116, https://doi.org/10.1210/er.2008-0033..
5. Richard J. Johnson, *Nature Wants Us to Be Fat: The Surprising Science Behind Why We Gain Weight and How We Can Prevent—and Reverse—It* (New York: BenBella Books, 2022).
6. Shu Wen Ng, Meghan M. Slining, and Barry M. Popkin, "The Healthy Weight Commitment Foundation Pledge," *American Journal of Preventive Medicine* 47, no. 4 (October 2014): 508–19, https://doi.org/10.1016/j.amepre.2014.05.029.
7. James W. Wheless, "History of the Ketogenic Diet," *Epilepsia* 49, no. s8 (November 4, 2008): 3–5, https://doi.org/10.1111/j.1528-1167.2008.01821.x; Kossoff et al. *The Ketogenic and Modified Atkins Diets: Treatments for Epilepsy and Other Disorders*, 6th ed (New York: Demos Health, 2020).
8. Satchidananda Panda, *The Circadian Code: Lose Weight, Supercharge Your Energy, and Transform Your Health from Morning to Midnight* (New York: Rodale Books, 2018); Pam R. Taub and Satchidananda Panda, "Time for Better Time-Restricted Eating Trials to Lessen the Burden of Metabolic Diseases," *Cell Reports Medicine* 3, no. 6 (June 2022): 100665, https://doi.org/10.1016/j.xcrm.2022.100665.
9. David A. Sinclair and Leonard Guarente, "Small-Molecule Allosteric Activators of Sirtuins," *Annual Review of Pharmacology and Toxicology* 54, no. 1 (October 16, 2013): 363–80, https://doi.org/10.1146/annurev-pharmtox-010611-134657.
10. Li et al., "The Effects of Daily Fasting Hours on Shaping Gut Microbiota in Mice," *BMC Microbiology* 20, no. 1 (March 24, 2020), https://doi.org/10.1186/s12866-020-01754-2.

Chapter 11

1. Srámek et al., "Human Physiological Responses to Immersion into Water of Different Temperatures," *European Journal of Applied Physiology* 81, no. 5 (February 11, 2000): 436–42, https://doi.org/10.1007/s004210050065.

2. Wilfredo López-Ojeda and Robin A. Hurley, "Cold-Water Immersion: Neurohormesis and Possible Implications for Clinical Neurosciences," *The Journal of Neuropsychiatry and Clinical Neurosciences* 36, no. 3 (July 10, 2024), https://doi.org/10.1176/appi.neuropsych.20240053.
3. Yankouskaya et al., "Short-Term Head-out Whole-Body Cold-Water Immersion Facilitates Positive Affect and Increases Interaction between Large-Scale Brain Networks," *Biology* 12, no. 2 (January 29, 2023): 211, https://doi.org/10.3390/biology12020211.
4. Andrew Huberman, "Using Deliberate Cold Exposure for Health and Performance," Huberman Lab, April 3, 2022, https://www.hubermanlab.com/episode/using-deliberate-cold-exposure-for-health-and-performance; Andrew Huberman, "Dr. Susanna Søberg: How to Use Cold and Heat Exposure to Improve Your Health," *Huberman Lab Podcast*, May 2, 2022, https://www.hubermanlab.com/episode/dr-susanna-soberg-how-to-use-cold-and-heat-exposure-to-improve-your-health.
5. Robert H. Lustig, *Fat Chance: Beating the Odds Against Sugar, Processed Food, Obesity, and Disease* (New York: Hudson Street Press, 2012).
6. Pontzer et al., "Daily Energy Expenditure Through the Human Life Course," *Science* 373, no. 6556 (August 13, 2021): 808–12, https://doi.org/10.1126/science.abe5017.
7. Narayan et al., "Lifetime Risk for Diabetes Mellitus in the United States," *JAMA* 290, no. 14 (October 8, 2003): 1884, https://doi.org/10.1001/jama.290.14.1884.; Robert H Eckel, Scott M Grundy, and Paul Z Zimmet, "The Metabolic Syndrome," *The Lancet* 365, no. 9468 (April 2005): 1415–28, https://doi.org/10.1016/s0140-6736(05)66378-7.

Chapter 12

1. Papaioannou et al., "Heat Therapy: An Ancient Concept Re-examined in the Era of Advanced Biomedical Technologies," *The Journal of Physiology* 594, no. 23 (December 1, 2016): 7141–42, https://doi.org/10.1113/jp273136.
2. Minna L Hannuksela and Samer Ellahham, "Benefits and Risks of Sauna Bathing," *The American Journal of Medicine* 110, no. 2 (February 2001): 118–26, https://doi.org/10.1016/s0002-9343(00)00671-9.
3. New Zealand Ministry for Primary Industries, "Livestock Numbers," *Stats NZ*, https://www.stats.govt.nz.
4. Laukkanen et al., "Association between Sauna Bathing and Fatal Cardiovascular and All-Cause Mortality Events," *JAMA Internal Medicine* 175, no. 4 (April 1, 2015): 542, https://doi.org/10.1001/jamainternmed.2014.8187.
5. Campanella et al., "Heat Shock Proteins in Alzheimer's Disease: Role and Targeting," *International Journal of Molecular Sciences* 19, no. 9 (September 1, 2018): 2603, https://doi.org/10.3390/ijms19092603.
6. Rhonda P. Patrick and Teresa L. Johnson, "Sauna Use as a Lifestyle Practice to Extend Healthspan," *Experimental Gerontology* 154 (October 2021): 111509, https://doi.org/10.1016/j.exger.2021.111509.
7. Hannuksela and Ellahham. "Benefits and Risks of Sauna Bathing."

Chapter 13

1. Nazik Elgaddal, Ellen A. Kramarow, and Cynthia Reuben, "Physical Activity Among Adults Aged 18 and Over: United States, 2020," Centers for Disease Control and Prevention, August 30, 2022, https://www.cdc.gov/nchs/products/databriefs/db443.htm.
2. "Physical Activity Guidelines for Americans, 2nd Edition," Physical Activity Guidelines for Americans, 2nd edition, 2018, https://odphp.health.gov

/healthypeople/tools-action/browse-evidence-based-resources/physical-activity-guidelines-americans-2nd-edition.

3. D.J. Wilkinson, M. Piasecki, and P.J. Atherton, "The Age-Related Loss of Skeletal Muscle Mass and Function: Measurement and Physiology of Muscle Fibre Atrophy and Muscle Fibre Loss in Humans," *Ageing Research Reviews* 47 (November 2018): 123–32, https://doi.org/10.1016/j.arr.2018.07.005.
4. Du et al., "Sarcopenia Is a Predictor of Outcomes in Very Elderly Patients Undergoing Emergency Surgery," *Surgery* 156, no. 3 (September 2014): 521–27, https://doi.org/10.1016/j.surg.2014.04.027.
5. Alice J. Sophia Fox, Asheesh Bedi, and Scott A. Rodeo, "The Basic Science of Articular Cartilage: Structure, Composition, and Function," *Sports Health: A Multidisciplinary Approach* 1, no. 6 (November 2, 2009): 461–68, https://doi.org/10.1177/1941738109350438.
6. Food and Agriculture Organization of the United Nations, "World Food and Agriculture – Statistical Yearbook 2023," Food and Agriculture Organization of the United Nations, 2023, https://openknowledge.fao.org/items/5c272dc7-e1b8-486a-b323-6babb174eee0.
7. Andrea C Buchholz and Dale A Schoeller, "Is a Calorie a Calorie?," *The American Journal of Clinical Nutrition* 79, no. 5 (May 2004): 899S-906S, https://doi.org/10.1093/ajcn/79.5.899s.; Klaas R Westerterp, "Diet Induced Thermogenesis," *Nutrition & Metabolism* 1, no. 1 (August 18, 2004), https://doi.org/10.1186/1743-7075-1-5.

Chapter 14

1. Charles M. Morin and Denise C. Jarrin, "Epidemiology of Insomnia: Prevalence, Course, Risk Factors, and Public Health Burden," *Sleep Medicine Clinics* 17, no. 2 (April 23, 2022): 173–91, https://doi.org/10.1016/j.jsmc.2022.03.003./
2. Harvey R Colten and Bruce M Altevogt, eds., "Extent and Health Consequences of Chronic Sleep Loss and Sleep Disorders," in *Sleep Disorders and Sleep Deprivation: An Unmet Public Health Problem* (Washington, D.C.: National Academies Press, 2006), https://doi.org/10.17226/11617.
3. Oliver Cameron Reddy and Ysbrand D. van der Werf, "The Sleeping Brain: Harnessing the Power of the Glymphatic System through Lifestyle Choices," *Brain Sciences* 10, no. 11 (November 17, 2020): 868, https://doi.org/10.3390/brainsci10110868.
4. "What Is Daylighting in Building? (Design & Criteria)," Layak Architect, https://layakarchitect.com/daylighting.
5. Holick et al., "Evaluation, Treatment, and Prevention of Vitamin D Deficiency: An Endocrine Society Clinical Practice Guideline," *The Journal of Clinical Endocrinology & Metabolism* 96, no. 7 (July 1, 2011): 1911–30, https://doi.org/10.1210/jc.2011-0385; Ross et al., "The 2011 Dietary Reference Intakes for Calcium and Vitamin D: What Dietetics Practitioners Need to Know," *Journal of the American Dietetic Association* 111, no. 4 (April 2011): 524–27, https://doi.org/10.1016/j.jada.2011.01.004.
6. Riley Black, "What Happened the Day a Giant, Dinosaur-Killing Asteroid Hit the Earth," *Smithsonian Magazine*, September 9, 2019, https://www.smithsonianmag.com/science-nature/dinosaur-killing-asteroid-impact-chicxulub-crater-timeline-destruction-180973075/.

Chapter 15

1. "Americans Now Check Their Phones 352 Times per Day," Asurion, n.d., https://www.asurion.com/connect/news/tech-usage; Tudor Cibean, "Adults

in the U.S. Check Their Phones 352 Times a Day on Average, 4x More Often Than in 2019," TechSpot, June 5, 2022, https://www.techspot.com/news/94828-adults-us-check-their-phones-352-times-day.html.

2. Nicholas Rizzo, "Over 50% of Americans Haven't Read a Book in the Past Year [2022 Study]," WordsRated, July 13, 2023, https://wordsrated.com/american-reading-habits-study/.
3. Linda Stone, "Beyond Simple Multi-Tasking: Continuous Partial Attention," Linda Stone, March 8, 2014, https://lindastone.net/2009/11/30/beyond-simple-multi-tasking-continuous-partial-attention/.
4. Mark et al. "The Cost of Interrupted Work: More Speed and Stress." *Proceedings of the SIGCHI Conference on Human Factors in Computing Systems* (2008): 107-110. https://doi.org/10.1145/1357054.1357072.; Kermit Pattison, "Worker, Interrupted: The Cost of Task Switching," Fast Company, July 28, 2008, https://www.fastcompany.com/944128/worker-interrupted-cost-task-switching.
5. Matthew A. Killingsworth and Daniel T. Gilbert, "A Wandering Mind Is an Unhappy Mind," *Science* 330, no. 6006 (November 12, 2010): 932, https://doi.org/10.1126/science.1192439.
6. Daniel Kahneman, "Daniel Kahneman: The Riddle of Experience vs. Memory," TED Talk, February 2010, https://www.ted.com/talks/daniel_kahneman_the_riddle_of_experience_vs_memory.
7. Patañjali, *The Yoga Sūtras of Patañjali: A New Edition, Translation, and Commentary with Insights from the Traditional Commentators*, trans. Edwin F. Bryant (New York: North Point Press, 2009).
8. Killingsworth and Gilbert. "A Wandering Mind Is an Unhappy Mind."
9. Thanissaro Bhikkhu, trans., "Ānāpānasati Sutta: Mindfulness of Breathing," dhammatalks.org, n.d., https://www.dhammatalks.org/suttas/MN/MN118.html.
10. Ven. Mahathera Nauyane Ariyadhamma, "Anapana Sati: Meditation on Breathing," Vipassana Fellowship, n.d., https://vipassana.com/meditation/anapanasati_meditation_on_breathing.html.
11. Wim Hof, *The Wim Hof Method: Activate Your Full Human Potential* (New York: Sounds True, 2020).
12. John A. Bargh and Tanya L. Chartrand, "The Unbearable Automaticity of Being," *American Psychologist* 54, no. 7 (July 1999): 462–79, https://doi.org/10.1037/0003-066x.54.7.462.

Chapter 16

1. Thomas Hübl and Julie Jordan Avritt, *Attuned: Practicing Interdependence to Heal Our Trauma—and Our World* (Boulder, CO: Sounds True, 2023).

Chapter 17

1. Mindy Levine, *Foaling Primer: A Comprehensive Guide for Horse Owners* (Lexington, KY: Eclipse Press, 2008).
2. Frank B. Gill, *Ornithology*. 3rd ed. (New York: W.H. Freeman and Company, 2007).
3. Linda Acredolo Moore and Susan Goodwyn, *Baby Minds: Brain-Building Games Your Baby Will Love* (New York: Bantam, 2000).
4. Donald Johanson and Blake Edgar, *From Lucy to Language* (New York: Simon & Schuster, 1996); Spoor et al., "Implications of New Early Homo Fossils from ILERET, East of Lake Turkana, Kenya," *Nature* 448, no. 7154 (August 9, 2007): 688–91, https://doi.org/10.1038/nature05986.
5. A. Gopher et al., "The Chronology of the Late Lower Paleolithic in the Levant Based on U–Th Ages of Speleothems from Qesem Cave, Israel," *Quaternary*

Geochronology 5, no. 6 (December 2010): 644–56, https://doi.org/10.1016/j.quageo.2010.03.003.

6. Kate Golembiewski, "How Chewing Shaped Human Evolution," The New York Times, August 17, 2022, https://www.nytimes.com/2022/08/17/science/chewing-human-evolution.html; van Casteren et al., "The Cost of Chewing: The Energetics and Evolutionary Significance of Mastication in Humans," *Science Advances* 8, no. 33 (August 17, 2022), https://doi.org/10.1126/sciadv.abn8351.
7. Karina Fonseca-Azevedo and Suzana Herculano-Houzel, "Metabolic Constraint Imposes Tradeoff between Body Size and Number of Brain Neurons in Human Evolution," *Proceedings of the National Academy of Sciences* 109, no. 45 (October 3, 2012): 18571–76, https://doi.org/10.1073/pnas.1206390109.
8. Michel A. Hofman, "Energy Metabolism, Brain Size and Longevity in Mammals," *The Quarterly Review of Biology* 58, no. 4 (December 1983): 495–512, https://doi.org/10.1086/413544; Richard W. Wrangham, *Catching Fire: How Cooking Made Us Human* (New York: Basic Books, 2009).
9. "Loneliness Statistics and Data 2023," Roots of Loneliness Project, *Rootsofloneliness.com*, 2023, https://www.rootsofloneliness.com/loneliness-statistics.
10. Veera Korhonen, "Average Size of Households in the U.S. 2023," Statista, July 5, 2024, https://www.statista.com/statistics/183648/average-size-of-households-in-the-us/.
11. Julianne Holt-Lunstad, Timothy B. Smith, and J. Bradley Layton, "Social Relationships and Mortality Risk: A Meta-Analytic Review," *PLoS Medicine* 7, no. 7 (July 27, 2010), https://doi.org/10.1371/journal.pmed.1000316.
12. Holt-Lunstad et al. "Loneliness and Social Isolation as Risk Factors for Mortality: A Meta-analytic Review," *Perspectives on Psychological Science* 10, no. 2 (March 11, 2015): 227-237, https://doi.org/10.1177/1745691614568352.
13. Rainer Maria Rilke, *Letters to a Young Poet*, trans. M.D. Herter Norton (New York, NY: Norton, 1993), 54–55.

Chapter 18

1. Dan Buettner, *The Blue Zones: Lessons for Living Longer from the People Who've Lived the Longest* (Washington, D.C.: National Geographic Society), 2008.
2. Jed W. Fahey, Yuesheng Zhang, and Paul Talalay, "Broccoli Sprouts: An Exceptionally Rich Source of Inducers of Enzymes That Protect against Chemical Carcinogens," *Proceedings of the National Academy of Sciences* 94, no. 19 (September 16, 1997): 10367–72, https://doi.org/10.1073/pnas.94.19.10367.
3. Helmut Sies, "Oxidative Stress: A Concept in Redox Biology and Medicine," *Redox Biology* 4 (April 2015): 180–83, https://doi.org/10.1016/j.redox.2015.01.002.
4. Valko et al., "Free Radicals and Antioxidants in Normal Physiological Functions and Human Disease," *The International Journal of Biochemistry & Cell Biology* 39, no. 1 (2007): 44–84. https://doi.org/10.1016/j.biocel.2006.07.001.
5. James Lind, *A Treatise of the Scurvy* (Edinburgh: Sands, Murray, and Cochran, 1753).; Kenneth J. Carpenter, *The History of Scurvy and Vitamin C* (Cambridge: Cambridge University Press), 1986.
6. Mohanty et al., "Glucose Challenge Stimulates Reactive Oxygen Species (ROS) Generation by Leucocytes," *Journal of Clinical Endocrinology & Metabolism* 85, no. 8 (August 1, 2000): 2970–73, https://doi.org/10.1210/jc.85.8.2970.

Chapter 19

1. Klepeis et al., "The National Human Activity Pattern Survey (NHAPS): A Resource for Assessing Exposure to Environmental Pollutants," *Journal of Exposure Science & Environmental Epidemiology* 11, no. 3 (July 26, 2001): 231–52, https://doi.org/10.1038/sj.jea.7500165.
2. United Nations Population Division, "Urban Population (% of Total Population)," World Bank Group, 2018, https://data.worldbank.org/indicator/SP.URB.TOTL.IN.ZS.
3. Manganaro et al., "Anatomy, Bony Pelvis and Lower Limb, Foot Joints," *StatPearls* (Treasure Island, FL: StatPearls Publishing) 2024, https://pubmed.ncbi.nlm.nih.gov/32491379/.
4. "Falls Are Leading Cause of Injury and Death in Older Americans," Centers for Disease Control and Prevention, *CDC.gov*, 2021, https://www.cdc.gov/homeandrecreationalsafety/falls/adultfalls.html.
5. Tess DiNapoli, "Global Shoe Waste: The Environmental Impact of Footwear," unsustainable, June 11, 2024, https://www.unsustainablemagazine.com/global-shoe-waste.
6. Victoria Rideout and Michael B. Robb, "The Common Sense Census: Media Use by Tweens and Teens," Common Sense Media, 2019, https://www.commonsensemedia.org/sites/default/files/research/report/2019-census-8-to-18-full-report-updated.pdf.; Monica Anderson and Jingjing Jiang, "Teens, Social Media and Technology 2018," Pew Research Center, May 31, 2018, https://www.pewresearch.org/internet/2018/05/31/teens-social-media-technology-2018/.
7. Valentin Magnon, Frédéric Dutheil, and Catherine Auxiette, "Sedentariness: A Need for a Definition," *Frontiers in Public Health* 6 (December 21, 2018), https://doi.org/10.3389/fpubh.2018.00372.
8. Ussery et al., "Joint Prevalence of Sitting Time and Leisure-Time Physical Activity among US Adults, 2015-2016," *JAMA* 320, no. 19 (November 20, 2018): 2036-2038, https://doi.org/10.1001/jama.2018.17797.
9. British Heart Foundation, "Are You Sitting Too Much?," British Heart Foundation, n.d., https://www.bhf.org.uk/informationsupport/heart-matters-magazine/activity/sitting-down.
10. Chevalier et al., "Earthing (Grounding) the Human Body Reduces Blood Viscosity—A Major Factor in Cardiovascular Disease," *Journal of Alternative and Complementary Medicine* 19, no. 2 (February 14, 2013): 102–10, https://doi.org/10.1089/acm.2011.0820.
11. James Oschman, Gaetan Chevalier, and Richard Brown, "The Effects of Grounding (Earthing) on Inflammation, the Immune Response, Wound Healing, and Prevention and Treatment of Chronic Inflammatory and Autoimmune Diseases," Journal of Inflammation Research 8 (March 2015): 83–96, https://doi.org/10.2147/jir.s69656.

Conclusion

1. "The Triumph of Science: The Incredible Story of Smallpox Eradication," National Foundation for Infectious Diseases, May 8, 2023, https://www.nfid.org/the-triumph-of-science-the-incredible-story-of-smallpox-eradication/.
2. John H. Taylor, *Death and the Afterlife in Ancient Egypt* (Chicago: University of Chicago Press), 2001.
3. Alan Watts, *The Tao of Philosophy: The Edited Transcripts* (Novato, CA: New World Library), 1995.
4. Alan Watts, *Eastern Wisdom, Modern Life: Collected Talks 1960-1969* (Novato, CA: New World Library), 2006.

INDEX

J

K

L

ABOUT THE AUTHORS

Jeff Krasno

I am the CEO and founder of Commune Media, a masterclass platform for well-being featuring the world's most renowned authors and teachers. As the rugged, if reluctant, face of the platform, I host the *Commune Podcast*, which features over 600 episodes and currently generates over 750,000 monthly downloads. On the show, I interview a wide variety of luminaries, from Andrew Huberman and Marianne Williamson to Matthew McConaughey and Gabor Maté. In addition, I pen a weekly "Commusing" 2,000-word essay exploring well-being, philosophy, and culture that is distributed to an e-mail list of over one million scattered souls.

The Commune brand animates in 4-D on a 10-acre retreat center and production facility in Topanga, California, where I host immersive events, book launches, and masterminds—including regular retreats where I lecture and lead participants through the protocols of my Good Stress program.

If there is a singular thread that weaves through the fabric of my life, it is the fostering of community. I am the co-creator of Wanderlust, a massively popular global series of wellness events that have been integral to popularizing the practice and principles of yoga in the U.S. and beyond. In 2016, I was selected by Oprah Winfrey to be part of the SuperSoul100 as one of the nation's leading entrepreneurs. Given who populates this list, I consider myself number 99 . . . but still.

My first book, eponymously titled *Wanderlust*, debuted in May 2015 and has sold more than 50,000 copies worldwide. I also curated the Wanderlust cookbook, *Find Your True Fork*, which came out in July 2017. In early 2021, I self-published a collection of essays under the title *Communion. Good Stress*, released in March 2025, is the book you are reading right now.

In 1988, I met my better three-quarters, Schuyler Grant, in art class. She has suffered me ever since. In recompense, I dutifully delivered her three X chromosomes who have now matured into unruly teenagers. God help me.

Schuyler Grant

I fell into relationship with my life partner and my life calling right around the same time, in 1988. I met Jeff Krasno freshman year of college. And I started down the path of vinyasa (or flow style) yoga around that same time, seeking tools to heal the chronic back pain that I'd been suffering since my early teens. It's been a long, winding road of intersection between the professional and the personal. Never easy, but also never dull!

I opened my first yoga studio, Kula Yoga Project, in 2002, just two blocks north of Ground Zero and two floors above Jeff's indie record label. Being a small part of helping NYC heal in the aftermath of 9/11 taught me the transformative power of in-person community. In a crazy endeavor to grow communal well-being to epic proportions, I helped Jeff bring Wanderlust to life. A decade of dragging our ever-expanding family from mountaintop weekend bacchanals to urban festivals followed, culminating in a move to Los Angeles to open Wanderlust Hollywood. Five years ago, we created a retreat and production property in Topanga Canyon.

Through 30 years of teaching yoga and mentoring teachers, I have developed a unique and beloved style of alignment-based vinyasa called Kula Flow. My advanced teacher training has minted hundreds of teachers and studio owners worldwide. I was also the creator of the 200- and 300-hour trainings for both Kula and Wanderlust. I am a regular contributor to the Commune platform, which hosts my diverse asana and breathwork courses. I am especially proud of Empowered Birth, a course I hosted and co-produced to support women's journeys through pregnancy, delivery, and postpartum (and which features some of the most intimate stories I've ever told publicly).

Though I now reside in Los Angeles, with my Jeff, our three daughters, and four chickens, I am exceedingly proud that Kula is still going strong across the country. I lead regular retreats and trainings, and I consider myself exceptionally lucky to still love vinyasa-style yoga—and the same man—after all these years.

www.onecommune.com

Hay House Titles of Related Interest

YOU CAN HEAL YOUR LIFE, the movie,
starring Louise Hay & Friends
(available as an online streaming video)
www.hayhouse.com/louise-movie

THE SHIFT, the movie,
starring Dr. Wayne W. Dyer
(available as an online streaming video)
www.hayhouse.com/the-shift-movie

***

BEYOND LONGEVITY: A Proven Plan for Healing Faster, Feeling Better, and Thriving at Any Age, by Jason Prall

BREATHE HOW YOU WANT TO FEEL: Your Breathing Tool Kit for Better Health, Restorative Sleep, and Deeper Connection, by Matteo Pistono

FAST LIKE A GIRL: A Woman's Guide to Using the Healing Power of Fasting to Burn Fat, Boost Energy, and Balance Hormones, by Dr. Mindy Pelz

POSTDIABETIC: An Easy-to-Follow 9-Week Guide to Reversing Prediabetes and Type 2 Diabetes, by Eric Edmeades and Rubén Ruiz, M.D.

SELF HELP: This Is Your Chance to Change Your Life,
by Gabrielle Bernstein

All of the above are available at your local bookstore,
or may be ordered by contacting Hay House (see next page).

***